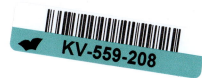

Payment and philanthropy in British healthcare, 1918–48

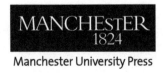

MANCHESTER
1824

Manchester University Press

SOCIAL HISTORIES OF MEDICINE

Series editors: David Cantor and Keir Waddington

Social Histories of Medicine is concerned with all aspects of health, illness and medicine, from prehistory to the present, in every part of the world. The series covers the circumstances that promote health or illness, the ways in which people experience and explain such conditions, and what, practically, they do about them. Practitioners of all approaches to health and healing come within its scope, as do their ideas, beliefs and practices, and the social, economic and cultural contexts in which they operate. Methodologically, the series welcomes relevant studies in social, economic, cultural and intellectual history, as well as approaches derived from other disciplines in the arts, sciences, social sciences and humanities. The series is a collaboration between Manchester University Press and the Society for the Social History of Medicine.

Payment and philanthropy in British healthcare, 1918–48

George Campbell Gosling

Manchester University Press

Published by Manchester University Press
Altrincham Street, Manchester M1 7JA

www.manchesteruniversitypress.co.uk

British Library Cataloguing-in-Publication Data
A catalogue record for this book is available from the British Library

Library of Congress Cataloging-in-Publication Data applied for

ISBN   978 1 5261 1432 7   hardback
ISBN   978 1 5261 1435 8   Open Access

First published 2017

An electronic version of this book is also available under a Creative Commons (CC-BY-NC-ND) licence. DOI: http://dx.doi.org/10.9760/MUPOA/9781526114358

Typeset in 11 on 12 pt Arno Pro Regular
by Toppan Best-set Premedia Limited
Printed in Great Britain
by CPI Group (UK) Ltd, Croydon CR0 4YY

Contents

List of figures

List of tables

Acknowledgements

I wrote this book in the hope of answering a question my Nan asked me over a decade ago. By the time I went to Bangor in North Wales to study History, I had already learnt her origin story. This had less to do with her childhood in St Werbrughs, a working-class neighbourhood in Bristol, or marrying a respectable Methodist scout leader, and more to do with his sudden, untimely death in the days following Christmas in 1965 – leaving her with two teenage daughters. After this she quickly began wearing trousers, learnt to drive and trained as a teacher. When I met her a couple of decades later, she was an impressive woman – a gifted educator, inspiringly self-taught on a vast range of subjects from world religions to art history, and who gave a mean rendition of '*Do Your Ears Hang Low?*'

When I returned from university and told her I was switching to joint honours with Social Policy, she asked me what that was. When I explained I was writing an essay on Lloyd George's introduction of health insurance as part of the National Insurance Act of 1911, her immediate response was to ask me a question. She told me of the 'dispensary ticket' system she remembered from her childhood. She recounted what was expected of her as a small child between the wars when her father was sick – walking from the east of Bristol to the city's north to go cap in hand to the vicar to get a ticket, then down into the city centre to the dispensary where the ticket could be cashed in for medicines, which then needed to be taken home. In total over six miles up and down some serious hills – a long journey for little legs. Why, she asked me, was this necessary? Why was there not a National Health Service so he could simply see a doctor?

In the time I've spent finding out and making sense of what I found, a great many people have been incredibly generous with their time and support. I would not have been studying History if not for my good friend Andrew Harman. The help of Steve King and John Stewart in setting up the research project was invaluable, and I am especially grateful to Glen O'Hara, Barry Doyle, Kate Bradley, Peter Grant, Roberta Bivins, Mathew Thomson and Pat Thane for their encouragement over the years. Despite common complaints about academia, I have always found my colleagues to be amazingly kind and giving people. The Voluntary Action History Society provided an especially useful intellectual home-from-home during my doctoral years. In the final stages, the Social History Society and my colleagues on the Cultural History of the NHS project at the University of Warwick have taken on this on this role. I am grateful to them all.

In conducting that research, the assistance of staff at numerous archives has been priceless. Amongst them, particular mention should go to the Bristol Record Office, the University of Bristol's Special Collections, and the staff at BCWA Healthcare (now part of Simply Health) who allowed me to rummage through boxes of the uncatalogued archive. I am especially grateful to the Bristol Reference Library, not only for their support in my research, but also for allowing me to use a number of photographs of items in their collection as illustrations in these pages.

Undertaking this work would simply not have been possible without the support of the Wellcome Trust. In particular, this book is based on the doctoral thesis written from the research conducted with the backing of a doctoral studentship (ref. 083402) and has been made available as an open access e-book thanks to further funding. It is no exaggeration to say I would not be in academia today if I had not received the backing of the Wellcome Trust.

The book itself took an unusual route to end up with Manchester University Press, but it has been a pleasure to work with Emma Brennan and her team. The advice of series editor Keir Waddington and the anonymous readers has also been hugely beneficial. I would like to thank them all for their thoughtful comments, which have always been based on a good understanding of my hopes for the book.

I have also benefited from the support of some wonderful friends along the way. Special mention should go to Jennie Maggs, Stephen

Soanes, Ceci Flinn, Clare Hickman and Richard Huzzey, for keeping me positive, grounded and laughing throughout. I'd also like to thank a father who taught me to question and a mother who taught me to care. Above all, the support of my wife Claire has helped me retain a sense of perspective and kept me smiling. Thank you.

Any errors are, of course, entirely my own.

Abbreviations

BCM	Bristol Council Minutes
BCWA	Bristol Contributory Welfare Association
BGH	Bristol General Hospital
BHC	Bristol Health Committee
BHF	Bristol Hospitals Fund
BMA	British Medical Association
BMICS	Bristol Medical Institutions Contributory Scheme
BRI	Bristol Royal Infirmary
BRO	Bristol Record Office
BSC	University of Bristol Special Collections
CBHI	Central Bureau of Hospital Information
COS	Charity Organisation Society
ENT	ear, nose and throat
HSA	Hospital Saving Association
IHA	Institute of Hospital Almoners
ILP	Independent Labour Party
LMA	London Metropolitan Archives
MOH	Medical Officer of Health
MRC	Modern Records Centre, University of Warwick
NHS	National Health Service
TNA	The National Archive
VHPPB	Voluntary Hospitals (Paying Patients) Bill

Introduction

In 1948 an animated public information film called *Your Very Good Health* explained the benefits of Britain's soon-to-be-introduced National Health Service (NHS).[1] It portrayed two different categories of hospital patient. The central character, Charley, says he is 'on the panel' as he cycles through an optimistic impression of a new town.[2] The narrator asks him to imagine that he fell off his bike: 'You'd be carted off in an ambulance, which might cost a couple of quid. And then you'd have to pay the hospital, too.' After he is convinced the new service will benefit him, Charley asks about 'old George up the road', who we first see walking past, wearing a bowler hat and carrying a brolly. When Charley asks him what would happen if he fell off a ladder he replies: 'I should call my doctor and have a private ward at the local hospital.' After the narrator describes the possibility of a series of specialist referrals and mounting payments, George is relieved and convinced that the new health service will benefit him too.

Why or how Charley would need to pay the hospital did not need explaining to a 1940s audience. Nor did the difference with the system under which George might incur mounting costs. Perhaps it was so ingrained in the everyday tapestry of British social life that it simply went without saying. The problem is that, looking back from the best part of a century later, we do not really know what went without saying. It is all too easy for those of us who have grown up with the NHS to anachronistically impose our own assumptions, either that things were the same or that they were different, onto the hospital system operating before 1948. We might assume that historians would be wise to this, but too often when they refer to payment in the pre-NHS hospitals they fall into precisely this trap. Although the abolition of payment became the most distinctive and widely recognised feature of the NHS, we never ask, or else take for granted, what the predecessor of a health service *free at the point of use* was, how it worked, or what it meant to hand over money to the doctor or the hospital.

For an explanation we can turn to Geoffrey Finlayson. Where Richard Titmuss observed that 'welfare systems … reflect the dominant cultural and political characteristics of their societies', Finlayson added that so too do 'studies of welfare systems'.[3] British historians living and writing in the era of the NHS have given questions of payment less attention than American historians, for whom payment and insurance are a daily reality.[4] The influence of a historian's context on the focus of their studies also explains the fact that British historians have increasingly started asking such questions since the turn of the century. By the time New Labour left office in 2010 it was the new rule that a 'patient's entitlement to NHS care should not be withdrawn as a result of purchasing additional care privately'.[5] This 'quiet revolution' meant that, in the words of a leader in *The Times*, 'the era of truly universal NHS care came to an end in principle as well as in practice'.[6] This direction of travel was followed apace under the Cameron governments. In 2013, the *British Medical Journal* reported that 89 per cent of NHS acute hospital trusts (119 out of 134) were offering private or 'self-funded' services and that private work in NHS hospitals was expanding.[7] Ahead of the 2015 general election, Conservative pollster Lord Ashcroft found mixed views on the NHS. Providing services free at the point of use was seen as its second most indispensable feature, after only emergency care, yet 50 per cent wanted the government to consider charging for some services.[8] What might those considerations be based upon? Fragmentation of NHS service provision has made it significantly harder for the government (or anyone else) to gather information about the situation on the ground, which leaves abstract theory or international comparison as the only options available – unless we look to the past.

This book does just that by examining the payment systems operating in British hospitals before the NHS. An overview of the British situation is given in chapter 1, locating the hospitals within both the domestic social and political context, before taking a wider international view. Chapter 2 sets up the city of Bristol as a case study to explore the operation and meaning of hospital payments on the ground. It places the hospitals firmly within the local networks of care, charity and public services, shaped by the economics and politics of a wealthy southern city. The options, obligations and experiences of Charley are considered in chapter 3 and then those of George in chapter 4; with particular attention to how the hospital payment schemes they would have navigated were introduced in our case study city. Treating the two in separate chapters reflects the distinction drawn between and separation of working-class and middle-class patients as a defining character-istic of the system that emerged over the early twentieth century. Chapter 5 will then step back to consider the social meaning of payment in such a system.

Essentially this book looks at four new arrivals in British hospitals from the late nineteenth century, each of which became commonplace in the interwar years. These were: patient payments, hospital almoners, hospital contributory schemes and middle-class patients. None of these were small changes, and the impact they had upon the philosophy of the hospitals is here recognised and characterised as a shift from a moral to an economic code of conduct. Yet it is argued that new systems of class division merely replaced old ones, ensuring such distinctions remained at the heart of the hospital system and serving to mitigate and mediate the rise of universalism in British healthcare.

Charity and change

There have only been three decades in British history (at the time of writing) when it was the norm for hospital patients to make some payment to the institution where they received treatment, those between the end of the First World War and the establishment of the National Health Service. Although fever hospitals and specialists were already admitting patients from across the classes in the final decades of the nineteenth century, many of those who could avoid hospitalisa-tion did so at almost any cost. While some institutions may have asked their non-pauper patients for a contribution and others may have pro-vided some services for a fee, the fact that most patients were poor ensured that payment was far from the norm until the 1920s.[9] Payment was then ended as standard practice in 1948 when admission and treat-ment mostly free at the point of delivery was guaranteed to all under the NHS.[10] In between we find the short history of commonplace hos-pital payments, which can be understood both as an effort to manage the transition from caring for the poor to treating the whole community, as well as an abandoned alternative to socialised medicine.

Institutional medical care before the NHS was provided by a complex and constantly evolving mixed economy of healthcare. This included various categories of public hospital, each for specific groups. Poor law infirmaries gradually broke away from the workhouse, while sanatoria were set up to quarantine and treat those with a range of infectious diseases. Although these public institutions provided most of the nation's hospital beds, and dominated those for the chronic and aged sick, it was only in the interwar years that local initiatives by the most progressive authorities gave way to a conversion of poor law infirmaries into community hospitals on a much wider scale.[11] The old practice of stripping voting rights away from those admitted to a workhouse on medical grounds was abolished in 1885 and poor law infirmaries became important providers of maternity care, which Lara Marks suggests had done much to lessen the stigma attached to them by the 1920s.[12] Yet, when taking over those same infirmaries in the 1930s, local politicians were all too aware that one of the big tasks facing them was to end the significant stigma that remained.[13] Alongside these public hospitals, most acute medical care was instead delivered in voluntary hospitals, despite the fact they accounted for only approximately one-quarter of hospital beds, with many of these clustered in the large teaching hospitals.[14] The voluntary hospitals were charities, often established in the eighteenth and nineteenth centuries, to care for the sick poor. They were 'voluntary' in the sense they were founded and supported by philanthropic donations, though funding from other sources including public grants was growing in the early twentieth century.[15] They were also entirely independent of the state as well as of each other. They ranged from elite and grand institutions linked to medical schools, where the pioneering treatments of the day were often tested, to small cottage hospitals, where local doctors dabbled in minor surgery. Across this diversity, the voluntary hospitals can only be understood on their own terms if they are understood as charities.

At the turn of the century there was only rarely any need for anyone who could afford their own treatment to enter either public or voluntary hospitals. Yet this was changing. When the Ministry of Health was established in 1919, a committee was set up to examine the changes taking place and what medical system would be needed as a consequence. The interim report the following year explained that the change was essentially down to advances in medical science and technology:

> In days gone by such conditions as appendicitis were treated with poultices and drugs in the patient's home. Now they are treated by operation, which is more effective, but requires more equipment, a team of workers, and a larger expenditure. Such conditions as diseases of the lungs formerly received clinical examination and treatment by drugs. They may now require, in addition, the attention of the pathologist and the radiologist. This means greater efficiency, but more organisation and higher cost.[16]

The early twentieth century was a time when medicine simply became able to do more and became far more dependent upon the technological capacity of the hospital. It saw considerable increases in demand for hospital admission, especially at the voluntary hospitals with their higher reputation. Yet hopes the new Ministry of Health would build a national network of new facilities to meet that demand were short-lived. Lloyd George's wartime coalition had been extended into peacetime, but became far less ambitious in domestic policy as Conservative voices calling for retrenchment came to dominate.[17] Instead, it was left to local health committees and individual institutions up and down the country to respond to and embrace the new era of hospital medicine. The four new arrivals in the hospitals can all be understood as the hospitals themselves seeking to adapt to and manage these changes.

Patient payments

One of the ways voluntary hospitals sought to diversify their funding, in the hope of increasing income to meet the challenges of the coming era of mass medicine, was by bringing in patient payment schemes.[18] This was not entirely new. The precedent had been set with the admission of private patients in London and occasionally elsewhere in the late nineteenth century, but the interwar years saw the establishment of payments for all categories of patient rolled out far more widely.[19] Their introduction may appear, upon first glance, to have ensured the voluntary hospitals at least were operating a system of private healthcare in the interwar years. However, we should not assume, simply because payment was involved, that this was a commercial arrangement. It is important to consider what payment actually meant in practice. Although the schemes varied from hospital to hospital, we can discern some typical features; three of which are especially relevant here. First, rather than covering medical services payment went towards the cost of maintenance, while the doctors continued to offer their services gratuitously. Rather than a 'medical fee', therefore, this should be understood more as a 'hospital boarding charge'. Second, at a typical rate of around one guinea per week (twenty-one shillings) for inpatients, payment covered less than one-third of the actual cost.[20] Far from being 'for profit' this was still heavily subsidised care. Third, a system of exemptions and reductions ensured payments were not a barrier to access. Pre-NHS hospital payments were less private medical fees and more a system of means-tested medical charity.

The Lady Almoner

The figure appointed to administer the new payment schemes was the Lady Almoner. Gradually between the 1930s and the 1960s the almoner would be rebranded as the medical social worker, but the original name is an allusion to dealing with money in the sense of distributing alms. The first hospital almoners were co-opted from the Charity Organisation Society, which sought to instil discipline in the Victorian world of philanthropy.[21] By the time of the NHS, the almoner was dealing with various aspects of after-care and social support that would fall into the fields today of not only social work, but also occupational health. However, the first appointment at the Royal Free Hospital in 1895, and others across the capital at the turn of the century, were focused on preventing abuse. In this case, 'abuse' meant the free admission and care of those who could afford to pay, and were not the intended recipients of medical charity.[22] Her job (as hospital almoners were almost always women) was not to decide who should receive treatment, but to determine the terms of admission. She could recommend people be sent instead to the workhouse if their circumstance was primarily one of poverty rather than sickness, or exclude those not poor enough for the hospital's charity, but usually her task was one of deciding what rate of payment to ask for. Even while at times resented, there is no real evidence the decision of the almoner or the request for financial contribution was resisted.

Hospital contributory schemes

There was an alternative to the almoner's assessment, with the questioning of a middle-class social worker and possibly a significant lump sum asked. Hospital contributory schemes were mutual societies which operated by taking a deduction of typically two or three pence per week from their members' wages; in return they paid any hospital fees for them if they were admitted.[23] Further definition can be somewhat elusive, not least because of their varied origins. Some developed out of charitable Hospital Saturday and Sunday collection funds, others were rooted in workplace collections, and in some cases one or more hospitals actually established schemes directly.[24] Schemes in different areas also adopted a wide variety of policies. For example, some schemes such as those in Newcastle and Glasgow pushed for an 'open door' policy, whereby once they had provided the funding, access was universal and treatment was free at the point of use. They bypassed the almoner system at an institutional rather than individual level and have thus often been seen as forerunners of the NHS.[25] Meanwhile, others adopted a style more like that of commercial insurance, including a range of additional benefits in either cash or kind.[26] While both contributory schemes and the almoner's assessment provided ways for working-class patients to make a financial contribution to the hospital, membership of a scheme did allow a degree of empowerment in how that contribution was managed.

Middle-class patients

A system of income limits barred middle-class patients from admission to the ordinary wards of the hospitals, but increasingly over the early twentieth century the voluntary hospitals and some public hospitals set aside space for those who could afford to pay, usually in a private room. The far higher charges for these private patients were not compulsory or adjusted in keeping with their circumstances, and an additional a fee would need to be negotiated with the doctor or surgeon. This is perhaps the area of hospital provision where we might expect the most growth, given the advances of medical science that increasingly made treatment in the home evermore unrealistic and the fact that, in difficult financial times, this was the only way in which hospitals could actually turn a profit. However, it appears that the voluntary hospitals were either unwilling or unable to exploit this attractive new market, with the medical profession often in favour of maintaining a division between private and hospital work. On the eve of the NHS, private beds only accounted for 7.2 per cent of those across Britain's voluntary hospitals. The lower level of private provision in the public hospitals, where there were more beds overall, is not so easy to identify. However, based on fragmentary statistical evidence discussed further in chapter 4, we can estimate that only 3 to 4 per cent of all hospital beds in Britain before the NHS were private beds for middle-class patients. As well as being limited in scale, private provision was heavily concentrated in the south of England. In the work of the hospitals, especially further away from London, middle-class patients remained marginal throughout the period.

Organising principles

Two core principles will be discussed as underpinning these four new arrivals in British hospitals. The first will be termed *economic reciprocalism*. This is essentially the notion that payment can be incorporated into the social dynamics of philanthropy, where there is always a social hierarchy of expectations involved. The gift can never be returned exactly, but demonstrations of religiosity, sobriety or deference might be elicited by way of reciprocity.[27] What is peculiar about the brand of reciprocity we find in the hospitals during this short period of three decades is that a patient's deservingness to receive free or philanthropically subsidised care could be demonstrated by means of paying their way, or at least being prepared to pay. There was a new financial focus, but the same dynamics of deference. Willingness to make a financial contribution became not only the mark of an appropriate recipient for medical charity, but in an age of mass hospitalisation it became the mark of a good citizen.

A combination of change and continuity also characterised the second principle of *class differentiation*. Where the hospital was previously a space for the middle and upper classes to fund and provide care for the sick poor, they too now might require hospital treatment. This might be expected to open up a new democratic era of in the social life of the hospital, but it did not. Instead, the separation of the classes and the provision of different services to each on a different basis became an internal event. The old divisions and distinctions were not so much brushed aside as brought within the hospital. Working-class and middle-class patients may have been more often treated within the same hospital, but it was only their medical or surgical treatment that was the same. They were accommodated in separate and very different settings, with their admission governed by very different arrangements.

All of this amounts to a period of dramatic change, yet those changes were based on a reformulation of the traditional philanthropic principles underpinning the voluntary hospitals. Payment was crucial to a reformulated brand of medical charity, but not its abandonment.

Notes

1 John Halas and Joy Batchelor, *Your Very Good Health* (Central Office of Information, 1948), http://film.wellcome.ac.uk:15151/mediaplayer.html? 0055-0000-4225-0115-0-0000-0000-0, accessed 25 April 2016.

2 When Charley says he is 'on the panel', this is a reference to the National Health Insurance system, introduced by David Lloyd George in 1911. It was a compulsory state insurance scheme for many industries, where contributions by workers, matched by their employers and the state, entitled them to be seen by a doctor chosen from a local panel. Only in cases of tuberculosis and some maternity benefits were hospital services covered.

3 Geoffrey Finlayson, *Citizen, State, and Social Welfare in Britain 1830–1990* (Oxford: Oxford University Press, 1994), p. 1.

4 Charles Rosenberg, *The Care of Strangers: The Rise of America's Hospital System* (New York: Johns Hopkins University Press, 1987), pp. 237–61; David Rosner, *A Once Charitable Enterprise: Hospitals and Health Care in Brooklyn and New York, 1885–1915* (Cambridge: Cambridge University Press, 1982), pp. 122–45; Paul Starr, *The Social Transformation of American Medicine* (New York: Basic Books, 1982), pp. 145–79.

5 Sir Bruce Keogh, 'Improving Access to Medicines for NHS Patients', 4 November 2008, 3, UK Government Web Archive, http://webarchive. nationalarchives.gov.uk/20130107105354/http://www.dh.gov.uk/prod_ consum_dh/groups/dh_digitalassets/documents/digitalasset/dh_ 090087.pdf, accessed 25 April 2016; Mike Richards, 'Improving Access to Medicines for NHS Patients' (Department of Health, November 2008), UK Government Web Archive, http://webarchive.nationalarchives.gov. uk/20130107105354/http://www.dh.gov.uk/prod_consum_dh/groups/ dh_digitalassets/@dh/@en/documents/digitalasset/dh_089952.pdf, accessed 25 April 2016.

6 'A Quiet Revolution: Co-Payments Are an Essential Part of the Future of the NHS', *The Times*, (5 November 2008).

7 Gareth Iacobucci, 'A Sixth of Hospitals in England Have Expanded Private Patient Options This Year, the BMJ Finds', *British Medical Journal*, 347 (17 July 2013), http://www.bmj.com/content/347/bmj.f4524, accessed 25 April 2016.

8 Michael Ashcroft, 'The People, the Parties and the NHS' (Lord Ashcroft Polls, January 2015), http://lordashcroftpolls.com/wp-content/uploads/2015/01/The-People-the-Parties-and-the-NHS-LORD-ASHCROFT-POLLS1.pdf, accessed 25 April 2016.

9 For examples of payment in nineteenth-century hospitals, see Jonathan Reinarz, *Health Care in Birmingham: The Birmingham Teaching Hospitals, 1779–1939* (Woodbridge: Boydell Press, 2014). On the limited payments taken in poor law hospitals, see Keir Waddington, 'Paying for the Sick Poor: Financing Medicine under the Victorian Poor Law: The Case of the Whitechapel Union, 1850–1900' in Martin Gorsky and Sally Sheard (eds), *Financing Medicine: The British Experience since 1750* (London: Routledge, 2006), pp. 100–1.

10 For the best concise introduction to the history of the NHS, see Charles Webster, *The National Health Service: A Political History*, 2nd revised ddition (Oxford: Oxford University Press, 2002).

11 For a fuller overview of these different areas of healthcare, see Steven Cherry, *Medical Services and the Hospital in Britain, 1860–1939* (Cambridge: Cambridge University Press, 1996), pp. 41–53.

12 Lara Marks, *Metropolitan Maternity: Maternal and Infant Welfare Service in Early Twentieth Century London* (Amsterdam: Rodopi, 1996), p. 198.

13 Bristol Record Office [hereafter BRO], Bristol Council Minutes [hereafter BCM], 1 January 1930, p. 250.

14 Robert Pinker, *English Hospital Statistics 1861–1938* (London: Heinemann, 1966), p. 2.

15 See Martin Gorsky, John Mohan and Martin Powell, 'The Financial Health of Voluntary Hospitals in Interwar Britain', *Economic History Review*, 55:3 (2002), 533–57.

16 Consultative Council on Medical and Allied Services, 'Interim Report on the Future Provision of Medical and Allied Services' (London: Ministry of Health, 1920), p. 5.

17 For critical and more sympathetic assessments of Lloyd George's postwar social reforms, see respectively Philip Abrams, 'The Failure of Social Reform: 1918–1920', *Past and Present*, 24:1 (1963), 43–64; Kenneth O. Morgan, *Consensus and Disunity: The Lloyd George Coalition Government 1918–1922* (Oxford: Clarendon Press, 1986).

18 For a discussion of this broader diversification, see Gorsky, Mohan and Powell, 'Financial Health'.
19 Keir Waddington, *Charity and the London Hospital, 1850–1898* (Woodbridge: Boydell Press, 2000), p. 87; Reinarz, *Health Care in Birmingham*.
20 Bristol Royal Infirmary [hereafter BRI], *Report for 1921*, p. 20.
21 Lynsey Cullen, 'The First Lady Almoner: The Appointment, Position, and Findings of Miss Mary Stewart at the Royal Free Hospital, 1895–99', *Journal of the History of Medicine and Allied Sciences*, 68: 4 (2013), 551–82.
22 See Keir Waddington, 'Unsuitable Cases: The Debate over Outpatient Admissions, the Medical Profession and Late-Victorian London Hospitals', *Medical History*, 42:1 (1998), 26–46.
23 For an introduction to the schemes, see Martin Gorsky, John Mohan and Tim Willis, *Mutualism and Health Care: British Hospital Contributory Schemes in the Twentieth Century* (Manchester: Manchester University Press, 2006).
24 *Ibid.*, pp. 19–43; Barry Doyle, 'Power and Accountability in the Voluntary Hospitals of Middlesbrough 1900–48', in Peter Shapely and Anne Borsay (eds), *Medicine, Charity and Mutual Aid: The Consumption of Health and Welfare, c.1550–1950* (Aldershot: Ashgate, 2006), pp. 207–24; Stephen Cherry, 'Hospital Saturday, Workplace Collections and Issues in Late Nineteenth-Century Hospital Funding', *Medical History*, 44:4 (2000), 461–88.
25 Gorsky, Mohan and Willis, *Mutualism and Health Care*, p. 139.
26 Steven Cherry, 'Accountability, Entitlement, and Control Issues and Voluntary Hospital Funding c1860–1939', *Social History of Medicine*, 9:2 (1996), 215–33.
27 Alan Kidd, 'Philanthropy and the "Social History Paradigm"', *Social History*, 2:2 (1996), 186–7.

1

Payment in the history of healthcare

'The voluntary hospital system is not dead', declared one delegate at the 1938 annual conference of the Incorporated Association of Hospital Officers; 'It may be changing, it may eventually become something other than a voluntary hospital system, but it is not dead.'[1] Ten years later it would be brought to an abrupt end, nationalised and integrated almost wholesale into the new health service. While this was undoubtedly a significant change in the organisation of healthcare in modern Britain, how to understand that change is open to debate. Historians and social scientists have variously understood the NHS as both a rejection and a culmination of what came before. These different narratives cast patient payment in contrasting roles. It was either an important indicator that the voluntary hospitals had effectively become private hospitals ahead of their nationalisation, or it was a major plank in the establishment of a more democratic form of health provision that prefigured a socialised health service. Thus, to appreciate the place of payment within the pre-NHS hospital system, it is important to understand the wider picture within which it emerged.

Payment becoming a standard feature of the hospital experience was not, however, an exclusively British phenomenon. After surveying some key themes in the historiography of healthcare in early twentieth-century Britain, this chapter will turn to a few enlightening international comparisons. Previous international perspectives on hospital funding have tended to focus on health insurance, which allows for some revealing comparisons. For example, under the National Health Insurance scheme British doctors were paid according to a rather ungenerous capitation fee, while the German system it was based upon had allowed the doctors to set their own fee for their service.[2] Equally, the French insurance system allowed patients the right to choose their doctor, whereas previously 'the so-called non-paying sick had had no such right because free medicine had been a charitable exchange'.[3] Neither British doctors nor patients were similarly empowered by state insurance and this comparison provides useful context for the patient payment schemes in Britain that likewise did little to empower either. In contextualising the British payment schemes we will focus on comparisons with the United States, France and Ireland. Each had a different experience of introducing patient payments. The American 'private patient revolution', the adoption of social insurance programmes in France and the distorting influence of the Irish Hospitals Sweepstake all contrasted sharply with the British experience.[4] At the same time, however, they each show the same fundamental changes to the technological capacities, social function and patient base of the hospital in the early twentieth century. Internationally and domestically, it is within this broader context, as one change at a time of many, that we can best understand the arrival of patient payments as normal practice within the British hospital in the decades preceding the inception of the NHS.

The road to 1948?

The establishment of a national health service was a key plank of Labour's postwar social reforms. At the end of the Second World War, business as usual was restored to British politics in a startlingly prompt manner. Only two weeks after the Allied victory in Europe, Churchill's national coalition partners withdrew their support and forced the first general election for a decade, and the first on traditional party lines since before the Wall Street Crash.[5] When Labour won a shock landslide victory, and the modest Clement Attlee took Churchill's place as Prime Minister even as fighting continued in the Pacific, some aspects of the new government's policy were characterised by continuity. The primacy of the Anglo-American alliance is the most obvious, but the wartime coalition had also been keen to follow the 1942 Beveridge Report in exploring the options for postwar social reconstruction. Beyond this, however, Labour's first majority government took Britain in a radical new direction.[6] Much of the empire was dismantled at an alarming pace while key industries including coal, steel, electricity and the railways were brought under state control.[7] Almost as an extension of this programme, Britain's entire hospital sector was nationalised. However, the creation of the NHS is usually seen as totemic not of Labour's nationalisation policies, but of its wider establishment of the welfare state.[8] While reforms to social security and pensions have little place in the popular memory of the 1945 Labour government, the NHS is often referred to interchangeably with the welfare state itself.

The hallmarks of this new health service were that it should be universal, comprehensive and free at the point of use. The funding for this came almost entirely from general taxation, breaking what link there was between paying for and receiving care in times of sickness. This was delivered by a tripartite system: regional boards for the newly nationalised hospitals, primary care services provided by self-employed professionals contracted to treat NHS patients (including dentists, opticians, pharmacists and general practitioners serving as gatekeepers to many other services), and local authority Medical Officers of Health overseeing the remaining public health and social care services (such as community clinics, health visitors for expectant and new mothers, school medical services and immunisation programmes).[9] Despite almost continual reform, this fundamental structure of the NHS has so far survived for many decades. There is, therefore, no escaping the significance of the 'appointed day', 5 July 1948, when this new health service came into being, three years to the day from Labour's surprise election victory.

For our purposes, we might see 1948 as the abolition of payment. Yet this clear-cut account needs nuancing for both before and after the introduction of the NHS. While questions of payment were removed from the doctor–patient relationship, it was only a few years before the very occasional payments for additional items were joined by standard charges for the services of opticians and dentists and then for all prescriptions. Meanwhile, the separation of private beds continued. Where before private beds had been the sole provision made for the middle classes, they were now able to enter the free public wards and amenity and pay beds became *options* for purchasing a greater degree of privacy or the services of a private doctor or surgeon. Indeed, the choice between free or fee-paying services meant the middle-class patient had more choice under the NHS than before.

Rejection or culmination?

With the transition from a diverse patchwork of providers to a comprehensive and universal service as the dominant teleological narrative in the history of British healthcare, change looms large. Yet there is no consensus on the cause, or even the chronological scope, of that change. Debate rages over whether the establishment of the NHS amounted to a rejection or a culmination of the developments of preceding years and decades. If and how payment is recognised as part of what came before makes a difference here.

The NHS itself, for its official historian Charles Webster, seems almost a fluke of history.[10] Aneurin Bevan, unexpectedly appointed Health Minister by Attlee, conducted what he calls an 'audacious campaign' crucial in determining the specific settlement brought about.[11] This gave greater prominence to central government than Labour's previous plans for a municipal-run health service, crafted in no small part by the Socialist Medical Association and championed around the cabinet table by Ernest Bevin.[12] While this accounts for the particular organisational form of the NHS, there is a good case that any minister from any party would have introduced a health service of some description. Indeed, to those involved with Bristol's voluntary hospitals, proposals put forward by Henry Willink, the Conservative health minister in Churchill's wartime coalition government, amounted to 'promises of free services for all when needed', which they feared would act as a disincentive to charitable support.[13] Whether Bevan is given the credit personally or not the narrative here is essentially one in which the NHS is ultimately a rejection of, in the familiar left-wing rallying cry, the bad old days of the 1930s – a refrain Bevan himself used in his famous speech describing those Conservatives he held responsible for the poverty he saw in his younger days as 'lower than vermin'; a speech given on the eve of the inception of the NHS. The complex realities of payment schemes are ignored in this narrative. Instead, payment exists as a symbol of free-market healthcare of a kind that in fact never existed on any significant scale. A more nuanced understanding of the place of payment in British hospitals before and after 1948 adds to a growing appreciation that it was the high-point in a longer period of kaleidoscopic change.

An alternative narrative has been increasingly favoured by historians, mostly since the turn of the century, whereby the new settlement of

1948 combated the serious shortcomings of earlier years less by over-turning all that had come before and more by universalising pioneering local initiatives. The wartime Emergency Medical Service has always been held up as an example of what could be achieved by a planned health service, prompting the British people to seek a more ambitious health policy,[14] but historians and social scientists have also started looking further back to find the developments of the interwar years bringing about some degree of co-ordination and integration.[15] While there were certainly pioneering municipal initiatives prefiguring the NHS, including the London County Council,[16] it is unclear how much the shift from poor law to municipal hospital provision actually led to any change on the ground.[17] Equally, historians have recently become increasingly aware of the voluntary provision of healthcare, and welfare more broadly, as part of a wider rediscovery of civil society in Britain's past. Moving beyond a whiggish view of increasing state intervention as an inevitable journey towards a better society, what Pat Thane has called 'the ruling paradigm of welfare state histories in the optimistic 1950s and 1960s',[18] has revealed a more significant role for voluntary hospitals and other voluntary organisations in interwar projects than might be assumed if progress is viewed simply as ever-greater state intervention on a march towards socialised medicine.[19]

This is one way in which it has been helpful for historians to distin-guish between progress made and steps taken towards the NHS specifi-cally. 'By looking at everything through the prism of the NHS' and measuring other systems constantly 'against the gold standard of some imagined NHS', Barry Doyle has warned, the risk is 'we overlook how far provision had travelled in the 20 years after 1918 and how much potential it had to continue to grow'.[20] Indeed, there were a number of viable alternatives to the specific form the NHS took. There is no need to make a judgement over whether any of these might have been preferable, but it is hard to truly understand the history of British healthcare without acknowledging that they existed. Some of these would have also provided medical care free at the point of use, whether under another model of public provision, with a mixed economy approach, or through the adoption of social insurance as a development of the hospital contributory schemes. Once we recognise the various options that were available and that some of them were already being implemented between the wars, what becomes clear is that any clear-cut distinction between before and after 1948 is likely to be an oversimplification.

This is true in the case of payment. While the interwar period's fledgling municipal hospital services anticipated the NHS in other ways, they also operated effectively the same payment system as the voluntary hospitals. Legislation in 1879 and 1885 had already empowered poor law guardians to recover 'the cost of maintenance' from those who were deemed able to contribute, although such contributions were minimal – amounting to only 1 per cent of income at the Whitechapel Workhouse in London.[21] The 1929 Local Government Act, passed by Health Minister Neville Chamberlain, both allowed local authorities to appropriate workhouse infirmaries as general hospitals for the community as a whole and required them to recoup whatever costs they could from their patients. As such, the interwar years offer a previously overlooked example of payment within a mix of public and voluntary hospitals as one of the roads not travelled. Just as there were no fixed or absolute boundaries between the various sectors of the mixed economy of healthcare, as Paul Weindling has noted taking a global view, the British pre-NHS situation demonstrates the practice of paying the hospital did not belong solely to one sector.[22] Payment may have been more common in the voluntary hospitals and it may therefore have prompted more fundamental questions of its traditional character, but it operated across the pre-NHS mixed economy of healthcare.

Hospital planning and funding: a local perspective

The approach taken here to investigate these payment schemes is to use, as a starting point for the analysis, the city of Bristol as a local case study. There are two possible reasons to adopt a local case study approach. First, to test out established patterns or explanations in a new locality. Second, to consider the local dimension of the issue under investigation when it is important to understand it fully. Our rationale is the latter. Indeed, the city has not been overlooked in the literature of pre-NHS healthcare. Martin Gorsky has assessed the city's 'haphazard journey towards an integrated hospital system' in the late 1930s, following 'several false starts' and disputes.[23] In general this was undoubtedly the case, with developments usually not co-ordinated between hospitals or sectors. Yet when it comes to the introduction and administration of hospital payment schemes, either in concert or in parallel, we find a perhaps surprising amount of uniformity between institutions, voluntary and municipal.

Indeed, the speed with which a common model of payment fell into place across British hospitals in the years following the First World War is noteworthy, not least because more generally this was a period in which a common model of hospital organisation was only established during the late 1930s. This is not to say that no earlier progress was made towards integrating local hospital services or that there were no previous pioneering efforts. Gorsky's work on Bristol is characteristic of a wider body of work, consisting in no small part of a substantial collection of local case studies, where a number of historians have sought to reassess the state organisation of pre-NHS healthcare. In his study of Manchester, John Pickstone suggested by the mid-1930s a local committee was doing much of the work that would later be done by the NHS Regional Hospital Board.[24] This was a notably more positive account than that offered by Richard Titmuss. Looking back in the first years of the NHS, he saw the problem not only as being that the voluntary and public hospital systems were so diverse, with differences between the two as well as within the 'multiplicity of individualistic voluntary hospitals' ranging from 'great teaching hospitals' to 'small, debt-ridden institutions', but also that they 'had grown up without a plan'.[25] While Pickstone was less damning, he also cautioned that in this respect Manchester was exceptional.

Perhaps inevitably there has been a focus on the pioneering exception. David Hamilton has characterised the Highlands and Islands Medical Service, established as early as 1912 and integrating general practitioners with other health and welfare institutions and services, as anticipating the NHS both 'by removing the cash nexus between the patient and doctor and by the comprehensiveness of its aims'.[26] The Bradford Municipal Hospital initiative of 1920 also serves as a good reminder that the earliest initiatives were not those of the capital.[27] By the 1930s, however, the London County Council was the largest single provider of hospital beds in Britain, and for some it offered a model of how local government might form the bedrock of future hospital reorganisation.[28] Indeed, one contemporary report noted that the area in and around the capital was a rarity for the 'comprehensive general public hospitals service' in development.[29]

Alongside these local initiatives were others under the leadership of the local Medical Officer of Health, to which Gorsky has drawn attention. One such scheme was the 'Aberdeen experiment', which he has described as a 'trail blazer' for its advanced medical-governmental-academic network.[30] Yet another example would be the ill-fated Gloucestershire scheme, covering Bristol. The scheme planned for a referral network of public and voluntary hospitals, health centre 'outstations' and contracted private GPs, all under the direction of the Medical Officer of Health. It proved too ambitious a scheme in an era of financial retrenchment in the mid-1920s and 1930s.[31] If public spending likewise meant that developments in the municipal field were subject to notable local variation,[32] Barry Doyle offered a positive account of the integration of public and voluntary hospital services in the northern industrial cities. While the story was not always one of the forward march of progress, he has found developments based on collaboration rather than competition from the 1920s to the 1940s bringing about integrated and rationalised hospital services in Middlesbrough, Leeds and Sheffield.[33]

These local case studies have done much to nuance the verdict on how successful or otherwise the pre-NHS hospital services were. They have slowly tilted the balance of opinion away from Charles Webster's view that competition rather than consensus drove what improvements were seen in the interwar years.[34] We might expect to find hospitals taking payment from patients bringing them into direct competition, yet, as the following chapters show, this was not typically what happened. On some occasions supposedly competing hospitals collaborated on the introduction of payment schemes, while on others a sense of rivalry may have led institutions to imitate such arrangements, but there is no evidence of outright competition for customers between local hospitals.

Hospital finance

One important strand within this historiography has been a focus on hospital funding. The history of the voluntary hospital system is itself, inevitably, bound up with funding. It was the emergence of a mass, industrial, increasingly urbanised society that brought about the conditions for its foundation. These were the capacity, demand and opportunity to tap the collective financial resources of the community through the investment of the wealthy. This drew upon an 'underlying ideology' Roy Porter saw behind the eighteenth-century hospitals, finding in their establishment an 'act of conspicuous, self-congratulatory, stage-managed *noblesse oblige*' evident in the wider Georgian moral economy.[35] It was through alliances of medical men, seeking to advantage their own professional standing and that of their given specialism, and their wealthy supporters that a second wave of voluntary hospitals was established in the nineteenth century.[36] Meanwhile, financial backing also came from local businessmen who saw advantages in the voluntary hospitals keeping their workforce patched up and treated in cases of acute disease.[37] Around the turn of the twentieth century, there was a diversification in voluntary hospital income, with new systems of contributory funding and patient payments being introduced.[38] In London's voluntary hospitals, Keir Waddington found declining income from invested income especially important for prompting the establishment of Hospital Saturday and Sunday collection funds towards the end of the nineteenth century.[39] At the same time in Birmingham, Jonathan Reinarz has suggested a democratisation of funding was seen with the growing importance of businesses and mass funding schemes.[40]

However, as the analysis by Martin Gorsky, John Mohan and Martin Powell suggests, it was not until the 1930s that philanthropy went from being 'a junior partner in the funding mix' into outright decline, and by the end of the decade patient payments were providing over one-eighth of voluntary hospital income.[41] They tentatively pose the explanation that the call for donations was undermined by the growth of hospital contributory schemes on one hand, and increased taxation to fund an expanding public hospital service on the other. Certainly this was a time of great change for public hospitals in terms of their governance, technical capacity, the range of services they offered and the demand for those services, as well as expenditure devoted to them. Alongside central and local state commitments to spending on public health, maternity and child welfare and poor law facilities, hospitals were becoming an important item in spending on municipal services.[42] Where public hospital services had been previously provided for sections of the community – paupers in the workhouse or sanatoria for infectious disease patients, for example – there was a move towards municipal hospital provision for the whole community.[43] Spending on this project exhibited marked variation depending on locality and the nature of local politics.[44] Yet one aspect of this complex picture that has gone almost entirely overlooked is the place of patient payments within the public hospitals' own funding mix, an issue to which we will return. Moreover, it is likely these changes in the growth of a public, tax-funded hospital system would have damaged calls for charitable donations to replicate many of their services. It would certainly be in keeping with the wider withdrawal of the middle classes from 'associational voluntarism' that Martin Daunton has suggested took place in the early twentieth century, resulting in a decline in 'the significance of philanthropic welfare' as 'a central element in the stabilization of urban society'.[45] On this basis it makes sense to equate funding success for the voluntary hospitals in this period with a move away from traditional philanthropic sources of income, as Steven Cherry has done.[46]

Recent work, however, has been less damning of hospital fundraising in the interwar years, not least Nick Hayes and Barry Doyle's examination of the finances of large voluntary hospitals in Leeds, Leicester, Nottingham and Sheffield. Where others have linked a democratisation of hospital governance to a move away from philanthropic funding, they see some of this democratisation taking place within the charitable support of hospitals. They note that fundraising became 'less dependent on elite contributions and much more located in those processes and activities where all members of society were encouraged to contribute time and money to generate common public resources'.[47] Central to this new, more democratic hospital fundraising was the public donation of gifts in kind, such as food or bedding, which significantly reduced the running costs of the hospitals.[48] Equally they have afforded greater prominence to the place of payment in their local case studies. For example, Doyle has suggested that what appear as substantial changes to the funding mix in voluntary hospital account books might actually mask greater continuities in charitable income and purpose. In particular, he notes that the growing revenue under the heading of patient payments in Leeds and of contributory schemes in Sheffield saw long-standing income simply relabelled.[49] Meanwhile, Hayes has highlighted the resistance to introducing new forms of patient payment in 1930s Nottingham. This included the forced resignation of the President of the Nottingham General Hospital, where replicating the middle-class private wards of the city's Eye Infirmary was amongst the unpopular changes he proposed.[50] As such, weaving considerations of patient payments into the financial and political analysis of local hospital histories is now the norm. We now need to take one step further and place patient payments centre stage.

In bringing the issue of patient payments more fully into this ongoing debate, it is essential to adopt a local approach, as decisions about the various systems and schemes of payment introduced were acutely local. There was no national mechanism for introducing a new hospital policy. Even after Lloyd George's coalition government established the Ministry of Health in 1919, there was no direct control over even the nation's public hospitals. The Ministry's limited influence was exerted a decade later when the Local Government Act made recovering what costs it could in payments from patients a condition of municipal appropriation of poor law workhouse infirmaries.[51] Yet it was a matter for the local health committee whether they wanted to opt for appropriation (only around half had done so another decade later) and then their responsibility to decide how and how strictly to implement patient payments. For the voluntary hospitals such decisions were entirely institutional ones. It is therefore vital to understand the institutional and local dynamics at play. At the same time, neither the issues faced nor the new approaches adopted were specific to any one locality. Thus we must place the local within its wider context.

The social role of the hospital: an international perspective

In response to these debates, a more nuanced analysis has developed around what types of funding continued or declined, a crucial aspect of the wider reassessment of the success or failure of the organisation and development of hospital services before the NHS. Our concern here, however, is not principally to contribute to this ongoing task, important though that is. Instead, our focus is on using those new mechanisms of funding to gain a better understanding of the changing character of British healthcare during this period. The question of whether a hospital could remain a charity whilst taking payments from patients, the recipients of that charity, is hard to separate from a wider historiographical debate in the social histories of medicine in Britain, Europe and North America, on whether the hospital had by now lost its social function.[52]

By the twentieth century, the very nature of the hospital was changing. Founded as religious refuges for the sick, they became modern centres of research and treatment as care gave way to cure.[53] The late nineteenth and early twentieth centuries were important years in a longer period of change, seen by Paul Starr as the moment of the hospital's 'scientific redemption'.[54] One consequence of this transition was that the traditional 'patient narrative' was lost in the medicalisation of the hospital, with the patient supposedly 'de-personalised' within the institution.[55] Moreover, the patient profile changed at the turn of the twentieth century, 'as rising faith in biomedicine, post-Pasteur, coupled with technological transformation made hospital admission attractive to the middle classes'.[56] Hilary Marland has rightly noted that, despite these changes, a 'multi-functionalism' combining the medical and welfare roles of the hospital survived into the twenty-first century.[57] To appreciate the extent to which the social role of the hospital has been maintained in Britain, it is important to recognise the uncoupling of decisions about admission from those concerning the terms of admission. The former became exclusively a medical matter while the latter continued to be mediated, mostly intimately by the almoner. This uncoupling also limited the impact of insurance and commercial arrangements on the patient contract. The contributory scheme voucher arrangements, Steven Cherry has suggested, brought about a 'quasi-insurance' system, radically different from the deferential philanthropic traditions of the voluntary hospitals, and effected the terms of admission but not admission itself.[58] In this way, admission was opened up while philanthropy was maintained in the relationship between the voluntary hospital and the patient.

Payment in American hospitals

This is a strikingly different account of the changes taking place in British hospitals to those historians have given for the hospitals of the United States of America, where many of the hospitals had been founded explicitly on the same lines as those in Britain. The largest of American hospitals were the municipal and county public hospitals relying on state funds and primarily treating the poor. While the elite voluntary hospitals were prestigious medical centres providing acute care, smaller religious and ethnic hospitals were less likely to be endowed and more likely to rely on patient fees. The smallest were the proprietary hospitals that served as private surgical centres for the middle and upper classes.[59] Across these institutions, fundamentally, the same categories of patient existed as in Britain, yet the change in the balance between them occurred at a speed and on a scale far greater than in the British case. As the twentieth century began, 'a new factor emerged, a vigorous crop of private and proprietary hospitals that competed for fee-paying patients with unabashed and unambiguous enthusiasm'. This, according to Charles Rosenberg, amounted to a 'private patient revolution' in the first two decades of the century.[60] This was not limited to any one part of the United States. For example, one voluntary hospital in Illinois was already evenly split between free and private patients in 1904, with four-fifths private by 1911.[61] Meanwhile, the oldest public hospital in Texas – founded in 1883 for 'only those citizens who could not afford the services of a private Doctor and hospitalization' – admitted private patients from 1915. They were consistently the majority of patients throughout the 1920s and 1930s, and by the 1950s represented over 60 per cent of patients.[62] Despite gradual growth up until their nationalisation in 1948, barely more than a dozen hospitals in all of Britain would have had such a high proportion of private patients. As Starr notes, since private rooms were usually for private patients the shift to private provision as the primary work of the American hospital was evident from changing architecture. 'General hospitals built before 1880 consisted almost entirely of wards, with only a few private rooms', whereas 'by 1908 large wards had declined to only twenty-eight percent of the beds in hospitals' and 'single rooms now accounted for nearly 40 percent'.[63] Meanwhile, in stark contrast to Britain, 'more proprietary than charitable hospitals were being built' in America at the beginning of the twentieth century.[64]

Starr explains the adoption of patient payments in terms of financial necessity, a direct response to the failure of donations and bequests to cover costs.[65] The dramatic rise of private patients in particular, however, he puts down primarily to the growth of surgical work, which 'provided the basis for expansion and profit in hospital care'.[66] Rosenberg has meanwhile pointed to a wider sets of factors: 'Hospital budgets, physicians' practice patterns, attitudes towards science, charity, and the prerogatives of class – as well as the x-ray, antiseptic surgery, and clinical laboratories – interacted to transform the early twentieth-century American hospital'.[67] Taking into consideration the broader range of factors identified in studies of US hospital finance helps to explain the difference with the British hospitals, which had the same core changes in hospital medicine to manage. Consequently some similarities can be seen; for example in the concerns about 'abuse' David Rosner has identified in New York, the response to which was a system of public grants that focused provision of independent charity hospitals on 'truly indigent clients' in the 1900s. This was a system that encouraged 'administrators to pay close attention to the payment capabilities of patients, to initiate means tests, and to differentiate services according to class'; and one which was policed by public inspectors charged with 'investigating doubtful cases', who we might understand as municipal almoners.[68] Even with this system, however, 24 per cent of patients in New York hospitals were private by 1921.[69] The American example is one of private medicine embraced by the hospitals, with an effect on their character. 'The rise of hospitals', Starr tells us, 'offers a study in the penetration of the market into the ideology and social relations of a precapitalist institution.'[70] Rosenberg likewise sees a 'fundamental shift in social function and world view' in the American hospitals.[71] The same has been charged of their British counterparts, yet with far less supporting evidence.

Payment in French hospitals

A different contrast can be seen from the French experience. France, like Britain and many other European countries, undertook wide-ranging health and social reforms after 1945, and as a consequence the interwar years are often dismissed by historians as merely a prelude.[72] Yet French healthcare in the period 1870 to 1940 has been described by Jean-Paul Domin as 'extensive'.[73] Over this period, numerous French cities constructed what Timothy B. Smith has termed local 'mini-welfare states', most notably Lyon and Paris, where the hospitals were transformed 'from refuges for the poor to medical establishments intent on catering for all but the wealthy' as part of an agenda to 'modernize and democratize'.[74] The means by which this was done was not through an American-style move to private medicine or a British-style diversification within a mixed economy, but primarily by turning to the state. The French system of hôpital and hospice allowed for a distinction between curable and incurable patients, similar to the patient base of voluntary and public hospitals in Britain, but both received central and local state funding and state direction to a far greater degree – and were consequently 'very clearly public institutions' in a way their British counterparts were not.[75] This was developed during interwar years, a time of 'quiet yet bustling reform at the local level' for French health and social services.[76] Local activity was combined with central reform in 1928 when legislation made mutual health insurance compulsory for one-third of the population.[77] Coverage began in 1930 and increased numerous times over the following decade, taking the proportion of the French population with health insurance from 6 per cent to a majority, and bringing a far greater degree of unity to the French healthcare system than the British.[78]

The system adopted in France was a different approach to tackling the same dilemma. With 1920s social insurance debates asking who should foot the bill for meeting the costs of medical inflation and bringing hospital medicine to the middle classes, there was a sense that the burden had fallen once again on 'the economic victims of the war': *the new poor* of smallholders, fixed-income pensioners and respectable but low-wage workers.[79] To cater for those not covered by assistance programmes, hospitals in Rouen developed a sliding scale system, where paying patients were admitted with charges between Fr5 and Fr15 depending on their circumstances.[80] That there was any demand for such a policy was a far cry from the situation 'prior to the interwar years' when 'a middle-class family would never have dreamt of sending an ill family member to the hospital'.[81] 'Hospitalization became a middle-class survival strategy' and lost its shame, Smith has suggested, seeing the cause as principally economic rather than due to advances in medical technology.[82] His overarching narrative is one of charitable institutions struggling financially and turning to the local state, who in turn looked to the central state, yet he also notes that in the 1930s financial need forced hospital bureaucrats to seek out private patients.[83] Barry Doyle has gone some way to uncover the wider history of private hospital provision in France. He found that France, like the United States and Britain, developed private provision in its public and charitable hospitals in the late nineteenth century. Unlike Britain, however, pay blocks in hospitals and smaller mutual surgical centres became common features of medical care in French cities before the First World War.[84]

Payment in Irish hospitals

One nation sometimes assumed to have embraced commercial hospital medicine more readily than Britain is Ireland. This is an important assumption to test, not least since Ireland only broke away from the United Kingdom to form the Irish Free State in 1922. As closely entwined as they were, Henry Burdett saw a difference in their hospital systems. In 1879, he claimed Dublin had 'done more to give the pay system a trial than any other town in the United Kingdom'.[85] Differences in relation to patient payment might then be simply regarded as one of a number of differences between British and Irish hospitals. For example, in Ireland the term 'voluntary hospital' typically referred to Protestant institutions, where Catholic voluntary hospitals might be known as 'religious hospitals'. They also operated alongside prominent public general hospitals, in the form of County Infirmaries, earlier than equivalent developments took place in Britain.[86]

Yet the differences in terms of patient payments come down primarily to the effects of a peculiar interwar episode of state intervention in Dublin. Across the rest of Ireland local variation falls well within the range seen between towns and cities across Britain. Contributory schemes were a significant factor in Belfast, in the northern area of Ireland that remained part of the United Kingdom, and which looked much like any major British city in this respect.[87] Meanwhile, the proportion of voluntary hospital beds for private middle-class patients across Ireland was only around 5 per cent in the 1930s, lower than that in Britain, catching up only as their paths diverged dramatically when Britain was readying to establish its National Health Service.[88] In 1936 the Irish Hospitals Commission described 'increased accommodation in General hospitals for that section of the community in a position to pay for it' as 'a development of comparatively recent times'.[89] The Bon Secours, a Catholic religious order, established a 105-bed private hospital in Cork in 1915 and another in Tralee in 1921. Some of the larger general voluntary hospitals in Dublin had opened private homes by the early 1920s, including a 100-bed development at St Vincent's and a smaller establishment at the Mater Hospital.[90] The Mercy Hospital in Cork had also established a private wing by the early 1930s. Prior to independence the Irish Catholic voluntary hospitals received no local authority funding, nor the Anglo-Irish charitable donations from which Protestant hospitals benefited. This was a significant factor in their nursing congregations becoming 'unlikely entrepreneurs' and catering for middle-class patients able to pay full medical fees and increasingly turning to hospitals for the most advanced medical care.[91]

The most notable factor, however, was the remoulding of the private hospital sector in Dublin in the 1930s, following the establishment of the Irish Hospitals Sweepstake.[92] This novel approach to fundraising, with tickets randomly assigned to horses in major races bought across Ireland and internationally, was a direct response to the financial difficulties of the Dublin voluntary hospitals. The responsibility for distributing the large sums raised fell to the new Irish Hospitals Commission, which soon found that in setting the criteria for eligibility to receive those funds it had an important new means by which the state could direct the development of the capital's hospitals. The 'guiding rules' they laid down made the balance between patients paying at different rates a condition of receiving sweepstake funds. This required 25 per cent of beds to be reserved for free patients and 20 per cent for those private patients who could afford to pay above the cost of their treatment and maintenance, leaving 55 per cent for those paying the cost of treatment and maintenance either in full or part. Meanwhile, the Commission stated in their first report that these guidelines should not be implemented too rigidly 'as to cause an implication that the provision, promptly, of facilities for all those who are unable to pay is not the overriding obligation'.[93] This was clearly an attempt to protect hospital provision for the poorest.

However, there appears to have been a problematic gap between voluntary hospital practices (the same in Ireland as in Britain in this respect) and the understanding of them underpinning the guidelines drawn up by Hospitals Commission. They defined 'free patients' as 'patients paying 10s. per week or less'.[94] Since it was not uncommon to find 25 per cent of patients being admitted entirely free, the guidelines actually allowed for a substantial increase in working-class payment. Meanwhile, the proportion of beds they said were to be set aside for private patients was five times higher than the rate across Ireland at the time.[95] While the specific mix of income from different levels of patient payment varied widely between the city's voluntary hospitals, the Hospital Commission's eligibility criteria unintentionally opened the door to a far greater scale of middle-class private treatment in Ireland's hospitals than had previously been the case.[96] This was perhaps the biggest contrast with the British voluntary hospitals, for whom slower and smaller changes were at the time, and have since been, grounds for seeing them as private hospitals in all but name.

Charity and citizenship

The criticism that voluntary hospitals, once taking payment from patients, had essentially become private hospitals should be understood as one episode in their longer history, in the writing of which their 'voluntary' nature has been a greater and lesser focus at different times. This was prominent in a wave of works examining the eighteenth- and nineteenth-century hospital as a site for the formation of middle-class identity.[97] To a lesser degree, the voluntary nature of the hospital was also significant for scholars asking what it meant to the poor of these centuries to be recipients of medical charity.[98] By the twentieth century, however, there is little place for such matters. The lack of attention paid to the meanings of class and charity in the literature implies an assumption that the charitable nature of the voluntary hospital was either undermined or entirely ended as it evolved 'from an institution reliant on the charity of the rich on behalf of the needy, to a service funded principally by its users'.[99] The increasing presence of private patients was described critically by Brian Abel-Smith as mixing 'trade with charity' and by John Pickstone as 'commercial medicine ... invading the hospital field'.[100] While others have challenged this depiction on the grounds that old sources of income were of continuing importance, we also need to question whether the difference between old and new sources of income really does amount to an end of philanthropy as the organising principle of the hospital.[101]

Central to this is the relationship between the institution and the patient. A philanthropic relationship does not, of course, depend solely upon the transfer of funds, nor does it carry any requirement for kindness. As Alan Kidd has noted, echoing the anthropological work of Marcel Mauss on *The Gift*, its hallmark is the use of imagined reciprocity (usually incapable of being enacted) to demonstrate and reinforce social hierarchies.[102] That philanthropy is defined by the donor and the volunteer, who decide the timing, scale, method and object of charity, is fundamental to this power relationship. By contrast, the passive recipient is afforded little scope for personal agency. This was summed up by Fernand Braudel as 'He who gives, dominates'.[103] Indeed, this view of the passive recipient of charity has much in common with the notion of the patient as a disempowered subject of what Foucault termed the 'medical gaze'.[104] Yet historians looking at the hospitals of the early twentieth century have tended not to see patients as defined by their powerlessness.

The interwar years saw a new consensus emerge, Gorsky has suggested, around 'the conception of hospital care as a right of citizenship'.[105] This would appear to foreshadow the thinking of sociologists such as T.H. Marshall and Richard Titmuss who looked to the welfare state to bring about the solidarity of a new communal citizenship based on 'class fusion'. While the NHS moved Britain's healthcare a long way towards this, it is hard to see the pre-NHS hospitals as embodying anything close to this social democratic collectivist ideal. Such a case could, however, be made for the voluntary hospitals' partners in the voluntary sector. The contributory schemes and medical aid societies certainly had stronger strands of the collectivist impulse than the hospitals. For example, Steven Thompson has described how in early twentieth-century South Wales medical aid societies attempted to provide 'comprehensive public services'.[106] Doyle has instead characterised interwar contributory schemes as an arena in which access and entitlement could be negotiated, as a means of ensuring what it was felt *should* have been guaranteed by right.[107] However, turning our focus to payment in the hospitals themselves encourages a view whereby the notions of citizenship embodied were not those of a passive recipient of welfare rights, let alone an empowered consumer demanding those rights, but rather an active one of a civic duty to financially support the system relied upon in times of sickness, yet with little control over the services provided. The pre-NHS citizen patient was therefore not so much a citizen-consumer or a welfare citizen as a citizen-contributor.

The social meaning of payment

To make sense of the fact that payment in Britain's pre-NHS hospitals brought about a new brand of citizen-contributor rather than empowered consumers, it is useful to briefly examine what has been said about the social function of money beyond the writings of historians. A long-standing and influential utilitarian notion about money is what Thomas Carlyle termed the 'cash nexus', according to which economic concerns and ties replace all others – social, cultural or moral. Following this line of thinking, Anthony Giddens described the dominance of money over social context as one of the disembedding mechanisms so crucial to modernity.[108] This view of money as a language that could communicate *value*, but was silent on *values*, has been challenged since the 1980s by scholars associated with the new economic sociology, such as Mark Granovetter and Viviana Zelizer.[109] Granovetter critiqued the treatment of people as atomised actors, even if acting according to internalised rules of behaviour, and called instead for a far greater focus on the immediate social context.[110] Especially significant here is Zelizer's work on 'earmarking', whereby 'the physical homogeneity of modern currency' obscures the 'different networks of social relations and systems of meaning' which served as 'invisible boundaries' to 'mark modern money, introducing controls, restrictions, and distinctions'. The consequent qualitative differences she identifies in the various payments found in everyday modern life – distinguishing 'a tribute from a donation, a wage from an honorarium, or an allowance from a salary' – remind us of the importance of adequately questioning how to categorise the monies that made their way from patients to hospitals.[111]

Yet these refinements in sociological thinking about money have made surprisingly little impact on historical study, even as historians present findings that resonate strongly with such ideas in works on topics ranging from the sale of slaves to the establishment of commercial trading networks.[112] Anne Digby did briefly consider payment as a form of social interaction, when she examined the 'financial dimension' that 'loomed large' in the historic relationship between a general practitioner and their patient before the NHS.[113] She found practices such as retrospective billing on 'the doctor's individual assessment' to place the physician in a position of great power, far from liberating the patient-consumer. Yet, at the same time, she noted that the British medical profession refrained from an American-style 'medical entrepreneurship' in the eighteenth and nineteenth centuries, something she attributed to 'professional custom and the prevailing gentlemanly ethic'.[114]

Despite such insights, it is those older utilitarian ideas about money that have unwittingly underpinned historians' limited considerations of the arrival of patient payment schemes in British hospitals in the early twentieth century. It has been assumed that, once money enters the relationship between individual and institution, existing values – those commonly associated with Victorian philanthropy – were swept away. The broadening of the patient base and the purchasing power of the patients themselves are assumed to have flattened the distinctions between classes and disentangled the delivery of medical treatment from a wider system of social interaction and even social control. The persistent assumption has been that the decades preceding the establishment of the NHS saw philanthropy neutralised within the arena of the hospital. As the following chapters will make clear, this simply did not happen.

Conclusion

The shift to patients paying the hospital has long been a feature, even if a rather minor one, of histories of modern healthcare. In the British case, it has served as an example of both what was wrong and what was already changing before the creation of the NHS in 1948. It has likewise been used as evidence in assessments of the ultimate success or failure of the pre-NHS hospital system. Only rarely, however, has it been considered on its own terms: as a pragmatic yet far-reaching change to the patient contract within a wider reconfiguration of the social function of the hospital. The following chapters will seek to address this, examining the workings, scale and meanings of paying the hospital in Britain during those final decades before the establishment of the NHS.

To do so, it is crucial to understand two defining characteristics of the pre-NHS hospital. First, for those institutions dominating the delivery of acute medical care, the hospital was a charity. The patient was not a medical consumer but a recipient of medical charity. This coloured the economic encounter that was brought about by the introduction of patient payments, setting a course not so much towards consumer empowerment as civic contribution. Second, whether in the voluntary or public sector, the hospital was a local institution. Although hospitals across the country showed remarkable consistency in the introduction of patient payments, decisions were taken at the local, municipal or institutional level. As such, the next chapter turns to our case study city, surveying the hospitals of Bristol and placing them firmly within a local economic, political and social context.

Notes

1 *Birmingham Post*, 7 January 1938.
2 Martin Gorsky, 'The Political Economy of Health Care in the Nineteenth and Twentieth Centuries' in Mark Jackson (ed.), *The Oxford Handbook*

of the History of Medicine (Oxford: Oxford University Press, 2011), p. 437.

3 Timothy B. Smith, *Creating the Welfare State in France, 1880–1940* (Montreal: McGill-Queen's University Press, 2003), p. 134.

4 Charles Rosenberg, *The Care of Strangers: The Rise of America's Hospital System* (New York: Johns Hopkins University Press, 1987), pp. 237–8.

5 Key texts on this period of British politics include Paul Addison, *The Road to 1945: British Politics and the Second World War*, revised edition (London: Pimlico, 1994); Harold Smith, *War and Social Change: British Society in the Second World War* (Manchester: Manchester University Press, 1986); Arthur Marwick, *Britain in the Century of Total War: War, Peace and Social Change, 1900–1967* (Harmondsworth: Penguin, 1970); David Kynaston, *Austerity Britain 1945–48: A World to Build* (London: Bloomsbury, 2007); Andrew Thorpe, *Parties at War: Political Organisation in Second World War Britain* (Oxford: Oxford University Press, 2009).

6 For rather different assessments of the 1945 Labour administration, see Kevin Jeffreys, *The Attlee Governments 1945–1951* (London: Longman, 1992); Correlli Barnett, *Barnett, The Lost Victory: British Dreams, British Realities, 1945–1950* (London: Pan Books, 1996).

7 For the wider literature on the 1945 election and Attlee's government see Addison, *Road to 1945*; Jim Tomlinson, *Democratic Socialism and Economic Policy: The Attlee Years, 1945–1951* (Cambridge: Cambridge University Press, 2002); Kenneth O. Morgan, *The People's Peace: British History 1945–1989* (Oxford: Oxford University Press, 1990), pp. 1–111.

8 See, for example, Rodney Lowe, *The Welfare State in Britain since 1945*, 3rd edition (London: Palgrave Macmillan, 2004); Nicholas Timmins, *The Five Giants: A Biography of the Welfare State*, Revised Edition (London: Harper Collins, 2001), pp. 101–39.

9 Geoffrey Rivett, *From Cradle to Grave: Fifty Years of the NHS* (London: King's Fund, 1997), pp. 30–1.

10 Charles Webster, *The Health Services since the War, Volume 1: Problems of Health Care, The National Health Service Before 1957* (London: HMSO, 1988), pp. 390–3; Charles Webster, *The National Health Service: A Political History*, 2nd revised edition (Oxford: Oxford University Press, 2002), p. 255. See also Charles Webster, 'Birth of a Dream: Bevan and the Architecture of the National Health Service' in Geoffrey Goodman (ed.), *The State of the Nation: The Political Legacy of Aneurin Bevan* (London: Victor Gollancz, 1997), pp. 106–27; Richard Titmuss, *Problems of Social Policy* (London: HMSO, 1950); Brian Abel-Smith, *The Hospitals 1800–1948* (London: Heinemann, 1964); Robert Pinker, *English Hospital Statistics 1861–1938* (London: Heinemann, 1966).

11   Webster, *Health Services*, p. 399. See also John Pater, *The Making of the National Health Service* (London: King's Fund, 1981), pp. 105–38.

12   See John Stewart, '"For a Healthy London": The Socialist Medical Association and the London County Council in the 1930s', *Medical History*, 42:4 (1997), 417–36; John Stewart, *The Battle for Health': A Political History of the Socialist Medical Association, 1930–51* (Aldershot: Ashgate, 1999); John Stewart, 'Ideology and Process in the Creation of the British National Health Service', *Journal of Policy History*, 14:1 (2002), 113–34.

13   Bristol and District Divisional Hospitals Council, *Report for 1944*, p. 3.

14   Webster, *Health Services*, pp. 22–3; John Mohan, *Planning, Markets and Hospitals* (London: Routledge, 2002), p. 10; Geoffrey Rivett, *The Development of the London Hospital System, 1823–1982* (London: King's Fund, 1982), http://www.nhshistory.net/Londonshospitals.htm, chapter on 'Emergency Medical Services, 1939–1948', accessed 25 April 2016. However, some of this narrative is called into question by the reassessment of public attitudes towards 1940s health reform in Nick Hayes, 'Did We Really Want a National Health Service? Hospitals, Patients and Public Opinions before 1948', *English Historical Review*, 128:526 (2012), 625–61.

15   See for example Martin Gorsky, '"Threshold of a New Era": The Development of an Integrated Hospital System in Northeast Scotland, 1900–1939', *Social History of Medicine*, 17:2 (2004), 247–67; Barry M. Doyle, 'Competition and Cooperation in Hospital Provision in Middlesbrough, 1918–1948', *Medical History*, 51:3 (2007), 337–56.

16   John Stewart, '"The Finest Municipal Hospital Service in the World"?: Contemporary Perceptions of the London County Council's Hospital Provision, 1929–1939', *Urban History*, 32:2 (2005), 327–44.

17   Martin Powell, 'An Expanding Service: Municipal Acute Medicine in the 1930s', *Twentieth Century British History*, 8:3 (1997), 334–57; Alysa Levene, 'Between Less Eligibility and the NHS: The Changing Place of Poor Law Hospitals in England and Wales, 1929–39', *Twentieth Century British History*, 20:3 (1997), 322–45.

18   Pat Thane, *Foundations of the Welfare State*, 2nd edition (Harlow: Longman, 1996), p. 277. See also Martin Daunton, 'Introduction' in Martin Daunton (ed.) *Charity, Self-Interest and Welfare in the English Past* (London: UCL Press, 1996), p. 1; Addison, *Road to 1945*. For a clear and concise introduction to approaching the history of welfare in this way, see John Stewart, 'The Mixed Economy of Welfare in Historical Context' in Martin Powell (ed.), *Understanding the Mixed Economy of Welfare* (Bristol: Policy Press, 2007), pp. 23–40.

19 Beyond the voluntary hospitals, see for example Linda Bryder, 'The King Edward VII Welsh National Memorial Association and Its Policy towards Tuberculosis, 19010–1948', *Welsh History Review*, 13:2 (1986), 194–216; F.K. Prochaska, *Philanthropy and the Hospitals of London: The King's Fund, 1897–1990* (Oxford: Clarendon Press, 1992).

20 Barry M. Doyle, 'Author's Response to Review of "The Politics of Hospital Provision in Early Twentieth-Century Britain"', *Reviews in History*, review no. 1733 (February 2015), www.history.ac.uk/reviews/review/1733, accessed 25 April 2016.

21 Keir Waddington, 'Paying for the Sick Poor: Financing Medicine under the Victorian Poor Law: The Case of the Whitechapel Union, 1850–1900', in Martin Gorsky and Sally Sheard (eds), *Financing Medicine: The British Experience since 1750* (London: Routledge, 2006), pp. 100–1.

22 Paul Weindling, 'Introduction' in Paul Weindling (ed.), *Healthcare in Private and Public from the Early Modern Period to 2000* (London: Routledge, 2015), p. 3.

23 Martin Gorsky, '"For the Treatment of Sick Persons of All Classes": The Transformation of Bristol's Hospital Services, 1918–1939' in Peter Wardley (ed.), *Bristol Historical Resource*, CD-ROM (Bristol: University of the West of England, 2001).

24 John Pickstone, *Medicine and Industrial Society: A History of Hospital Development in Manchester and Its Region* (Manchester: Manchester University Press, 1985), p. 272.

25 Titmuss, *Problems of Social Policy*, pp. 66–7.

26 David Hamilton, 'The Highlands and Islands Medical Service' in Gordon McLachlan (ed.), *Improving the Common Weal: Aspects of Scottish Health Services 1900–1984* (Edinburgh: Edinburgh University Press, 1987), p. 483.

27 Tim Willis, 'The Bradford Municipal Hospital Experiment of 1920: The Emergence of the Mixed Economy in Hospital Provision in Inter-War Britain' in Gorsky and Sheard (eds), *Financing Medicine*, pp. 130–44.

28 Stewart, 'Finest Municipal Hospital Service'.

29 Political and Economic Planning, 'Report on the British Health Services' (London: PEP, 1937), p. 17.

30 Gorsky, 'Threshold of a New Era', pp. 249 and 265.

31 Martin Gorsky, 'The Gloucestershire Extension of Medical Services Scheme: An Experiment in the Integration of Health Services in Britain before the NHS', *Medical History*, 50:4 (2006), 510.

32 Alysa Levene, Martin Powell, John Stewart and Becky Taylor, *From Cradle to Grave: Municipal Provision in Interwar England and Wales* (Bern: Peter Lang, 2011).

33 Barry Doyle, 'Power and Accountability in the Voluntary Hospitals of Middlesbrough 1900–48' in Peter Shapely and Anne Borsay (eds), *Medicine, Charity and Mutual Aid: The Consumption of Health and Welfare, c.1550–1950* (Aldershot: Ashgate, 2006), pp. 207–24; Barry M. Doyle, *The Politics of Hospital Provision in Early 20th-Century Britain* (London: Pickering and Chatto, 2014).

34 Charles Webster, 'Conflict and Consensus: Explaining the British Health Service', *Twentieth Century British History*, 1:2 (1990), 115–51.

35 Roy Porter, 'The Gift Relation: Philanthropy and Provincial Hospitals in Eighteenth-Century England' in Lindsay Granshaw and Roy Porter (eds), *The Hospital in History* (London: Routledge, 1989), pp. 150–2. On the early history of the voluntary hospitals, see John Woodward, *To Do the Sick No Harm: A Study of the British Voluntary Hospital System to 1875* (London: Routledge and Kegan Paul, 1974).

36 Lindsay Granshaw, ' "Fame and Fortune by Means of Bricks and Mortar": The Medical Profession and Specialist Hospitals in Britain, 1800–1948' in Granshaw and Porter (eds), *Hospital in History*, pp. 199–220.

37 Hilary Marland, 'Lay and Medical Conceptions of Medical Charity during the Nineteenth Century' in Jonathan Barry and Colin Jones (eds), *Medicine and Charity before the Welfare State* (London: Routledge, 1991), pp. 149–71.

38 Jonathan Reinarz, 'Investigating the "deserving" Poor: Charity, Discipline and Voluntary Hospitals in Nineteenth-Century Birmingham' in Shapely and Borsay (eds), *Medicine, Charity and Mutual Aid*, pp. 111–33; Martin Gorsky, John Mohan, and Martin Powell, 'British Voluntary Hospitals 1871–1939: The Geography of Provision and Utilization', *Journal of Historical Geography*, 25:4 (1999), 476.

39 Keir Waddington, ' "Grasping Gratitude": Charity and Hospital Finance in Late-Victorian London' in Daunton (ed.), *Charity, Self-Interest*, pp. 181–202.

40 Jonathan Reinarz, 'Charitable Bodies: The Funding of Birmingham's Voluntary Hospitals in the Nineteenth Century' in Gorsky and Sheard (eds), *Financing Medicine*, pp. 40–58.

41 Martin Gorsky, John Mohan and Martin Powell, 'The Financial Health of Voluntary Hospitals in Interwar Britain', *Economic History Review*, 55:3 (2002), 549–50.

42 Martin Gorsky and Sally Sheard, 'Introduction' in Gorsky and Sheard (eds), *Financing Medicine*, pp. 9–10.

43 Powell, 'An Expanding Service'; George Campbell Gosling and Stephen Soanes, 'Healthcare and the Community in Modern Britain', *Family and Community History*, 12:2 (2009), 101–6.

44 For an extensive discussion, see Levene *et al.*, *Cradle to Grave*.

45 Martin Daunton, 'Payment and Participation: Welfare and State-Formation in Britain, 1990–1951', *Past and Present*, 150 (1990), 188–91.

46 Steven Cherry, 'Before the National Health Service: Financing the Voluntary Hospitals, 1900–1939', *Economic History Review*, 50:2 (1997), 305–26.

47 Nick Hayes and Barry M. Doyle, 'Eggs, Rags and Whist Drives: Popular Munificence and the Development of Provincial Medical Voluntarism between the Wars', *Historical Research*, 86:234 (2013), 714.

48 *Ibid.*, 734–7.

49 Doyle, *Politics of Hospital Provision*, p. 136.

50 Nick Hayes, '"Our Hospitals"? Voluntary Provision, Community and Civic Consciousness in Nottingham Before the NHS', *Midland History*, 37:1 (2012), 100.

51 See Alysa Levene, Martin Powell, and John Stewart, 'Patterns of Municipal Health Expenditure in Interwar England and Wales', *Bulletin of the History of Medicine*, 78:3 (2004), 644–6.

52 For a good introduction to the changing social function of the hospital, see Hilary Marland, 'The Changing Role of the Hospital, 1800–1900' in Deborah Brunton (ed.), *Medicine Transformed: Health, Disease and Society in Europe 1800–1930* (Manchester: Manchester University Press, 2004), pp. 31–60.

53 On the long history of the hospital see, for example, Guenter Risse, *Mending Bodies, Saving Souls: A History of Hospitals* (Oxford: Oxford University Press, 1999).

54 Paul Starr, *The Social Transformation of American Medicine* (New York: Basic Books, 1982), p. 145.

55 On the patient narrative see, for example, Mary Fissell, 'The Disappearance of the Patient Narrative and the Invention of Hospital Medicine' in Roger French and Andrew Wear (eds), *British Medicine in an Age of Reform* (London: Routledge, 2002), pp. 92–109. On 'de-personalisation' see Reinarz, 'Investigating the Deserving Poor'; Reinarz, 'Charitable Bodies'.

56 Gorsky, 'Political Economy', p. 435.

57 Marland, 'Changing Role of the Hospital', p. 58.

58 Steven Cherry, 'Beyond National Health Insurance. The Voluntary Hospitals and Hospital Contributory Schemes: A Regional Study', *Social History of Medicine*, 5:3 (1992), 455–82.

59 Starr, *Social Transformation*, p. 171.

60 Rosenberg, *Care of Strangers*, pp. 237–8.

61 James Monahan, *Bear Ye One Another's Burdens: The Growth of Rockford Memorial Hospital, 1900–1983* (Rockford, Illinois, 1985), p. 10.

62 Austin History Center, H2700 (1): Brackenridge Hospital, History and Description (folder 2), *The Good Life in Austin: A Brief History of Brackenridge Hospital* (loose pages).
63 Starr, *Social Transformation*, p. 159.
64 *Ibid.*, p. 165.
65 *Ibid.*, p. 154.
66 *Ibid.*, p. 157.
67 Rosenberg, *Care of Strangers*, p. 237.
68 David Rosner, *A Once Charitable Enterprise: Hospitals and Health Care in Brooklyn and New York, 1885–1915* (Cambridge: Cambridge University Press, 1982), pp. 138–49.
69 Rosenberg, *Care of Strangers*, p. 161.
70 Starr, *Social Transformation*, p. 148.
71 Rosenberg, *Care of Strangers*, p. 253. For the general discussion on this point see pp. 252–8.
72 Richard Freeman, *The Politics of Health in Europe* (Manchester: Manchester University Press, 2000), pp. 14–23.
73 Jean-Paul Domin, *Une Histoire Economique de l'Hôpital (XIXe–XXe Siècles): Une Analyse Rétrospective du Développement Hospitalier*, 2 vols (Paris: La Documentation Française, 2008) cited in Barry M. Doyle, 'Healthcare before Welfare States: Hospitals in Early Twentieth Century England and France', *Canadian Bulletin of Medical History*, 33:1 (2016), 174–204.
74 Timothy B. Smith, *Creating the Welfare State in France, 1880–1940* (Montreal: McGill-Queen's University Press, 2003), pp. 3 and 115.
75 For an overview of the French hospital system and comparison with the British, see Doyle, 'Healthcare before Welfare States'.
76 Smith, *Creating the Welfare State*, pp. 94–5.
77 *Ibid.*, pp. 98–9; Gorsky, 'Political Economy', p. 437.
78 Smith, *Creating the Welfare State*, pp. 132–4.
79 *Ibid.*, pp. 125–30.
80 *Ibid.*, p. 128.
81 *Ibid.*, p. 153.
82 *Ibid.*, p. 154.
83 *Ibid.*, pp. 129 and 152.
84 Doyle, 'Healthcare before Welfare States'.
85 Henry Burdett, *Pay Hospitals and Paying Wards throughout the World: Facts in Support of a Re-Arrangement of the English System of Medical Relief* (London: J.&A. Churchill, 1879), p. 93.
86 For an introduction to the various healthcare services operating in Ireland historically, see Ruth Barrington, *Health, Medicine and Politics in Ireland, 1900–1970* (Institute of Public Administration: Dublin, 1987).

87 Donnacha Seán Lucey and George Campbell Gosling, 'Paying for Health: Comparative Perspectives on Patient Payment and Contributions for Hospital Provision in Ireland' in Donnacha Seán Lucey and Virginia Crossman (eds), *Healthcare in Ireland and Britain from 1850: Voluntary, Regional and Comparative Perspectives* (London: Institute of Historical Research, 2015), pp. 81–92.

88 *Hospitals Year-Books* (London: Central Bureau of Hospital Information [hereafter CBHI], 1933–1947).

89 Hospital Commission, *First General Report, 1933–34* (Dublin, 1936), p. 68.

90 *Ibid.*, pp. 16 and 122.

91 Lucey and Gosling, 'Paying for Health', p. 94.

92 Marie Coleman, *The Irish Sweep: A History of the Irish Hospitals Sweepstakes, 1930–87* (Dublin: University College Dublin Press, 2009).

93 Hospital Commission, *First Report*, p. 69.

94 *Ibid.*

95 *Hospitals Year-Book* (London: CBHI, 1933).

96 See Lucey and Gosling, 'Paying for Health', pp. 92–9.

97 Hilary Marland, *Medicine and Society in Wakefield and Huddersfield, 1780–1870* (Cambridge: Cambridge University Press, 1987); R.J. Morris, *Class, Sect and Party. The Making of the British Middle Class: Leeds, 1820–50* (Manchester: Manchester University Press, 1990); Martin Gorsky, *Patterns of Philanthropy: Charity and Society in Nineteenth-Century Bristol* (Woodbridge: Boydell & Brewer Ltd, 1999).

98 Mary Fissell, *Patients, Power, and the Poor in Eighteenth-Century Bristol* (Cambridge: Cambridge University Press, 1991); Gorsky, *Patterns of Philanthropy*.

99 Gorsky and Sheard, 'Introduction', p. 2.

100 Abel-Smith, *Hospitals*, p. 338; Pickstone, *Medicine and Industrial Society*, p. 259.

101 For work that does focus on the continuing importance of traditional sources of philanthropic income, see Hayes and Doyle, 'Eggs, Rags and Whist Drives'.

102 See Alan Kidd, 'Philanthropy and the "Social History Paradigm"', *Social History*, 2:2 (1996), 180. See also Marcel Mauss, *The Gift* (London: Routledge, 1990) [originally published 1950].

103 Fernand Braudel, *The Mediterranean and the Mediterranean World in the Age of Philip II, Volume 2*, 1996 edition (Berkeley: University of California Press, 1949), p. 826.

104 Michel Foucault, *The Birth of the Clinic: An Archaeology of Medical Perception* (London: Tavistock Publications, 1973).

105 Gorsky, 'Transformation of Bristol's Hospital Services'.
106 Steven Thompson, 'A Proletarian Public Sphere: Working-Class Provision of Medical Services and Care in South Wales, c.1900–1948' in Anne Borsay (ed.), *Medicine in Wales c.1800–2000: Public Service or Private Commodity?* (Cardiff: University of Wales Press, 2003), p. 87.
107 Doyle, 'Politics of Voluntary Care'; Barry M. Doyle, 'Labour and Hospitals in Three Yorkshire Towns: Middlesbrough, Leeds, Sheffield, 1919–1938', *Social History of Medicine*, 23:2 (2010), 374–92.
108 Anthony Giddens, *The Consequences of Modernity* (Stanford: Stanford University Press, 1990), pp. 21–5.
109 See Geoffrey Ingham, *The Nature of Money* (Cambridge: Polity, 2004), especially ch. 3: 'Money in Sociological Theory'.
110 Mark Granovetter, 'Economic Action and Social Structure: The Problem of Embeddedness', *American Journal of Sociology*, 91:3 (1985), 482.
111 On 'earmarking' see Viviana A. Zelizer, *The Social Meaning of Money: Pin Money, Paychecks, Poor Relief, and Other Currencies* (New York: Princeton University Press, 1994), pp. 21–5.
112 See, for example, Dea Boster, *African American Slavery and Disability: Bodies, Property and Power in the Antebellum South, 1800–1860* (London: Routledge, 2013) and Sheryllynne Haggerty, *'Merely for Money'? Business Culture in the British Atlantic, 1750–1815* (Liverpool: Liverpool University Press, 2012).
113 Anne Digby, *The Evolution of British General Practice, 1850–1948* (Oxford: Oxford University Press, 1999), p. 242.
114 *Ibid.*, p. 94; Anne Digby, *Making a Medical Living: Doctors and Patients in the English Market for Medicine, 1720–1911* (Cambridge: Cambridge University Press, 1994), p. 135.

2

Medicine and charity in Bristol

Before the NHS, British healthcare had no national system.[1] While policies could be agreed and pursued by the Ministry of Health, the British Medical Association (BMA), the Institute of Hospital Almoners or any other national body, decision-making was distinctly local. For public hospitals this meant either the poor law union or the municipal authority. In the voluntary hospital sector, it was institutional. It is therefore only through investigation at the level of the hospital itself that we can really hope to gain insight into the uncomfortable accommodation between payment and philanthropy that emerged in the early twentieth century. As sites of charity, sites of care and sites of decision-making, these institutions were independent, although they did not operate in isolation. Context is important, and this means understanding the local economic, political and social context as well as the health and welfare sector within which the hospital operated.

Our case study is the city of Bristol, sitting within the historic county of Gloucestershire, on the border with Somerset, in the South West of England (see figure 2.1). In the mid-eighteenth century this port city, although slightly smaller than Edinburgh and far smaller than London, had been the largest of England's provincial towns and cities, before the rapid growth of manufacturing centres in the Midlands and the North. While the early twentieth century saw Birmingham overtake Liverpool and Manchester to become England's second most populous city behind London, Bristol's steady growth has seen it remain seventh from the mid-nineteenth century behind Leeds and Sheffield; smaller than the major Scottish cities of Glasgow and Edinburgh but larger than nearby Cardiff or any other Welsh city.[2] The importance of Bristol lies less in its role as regional centre

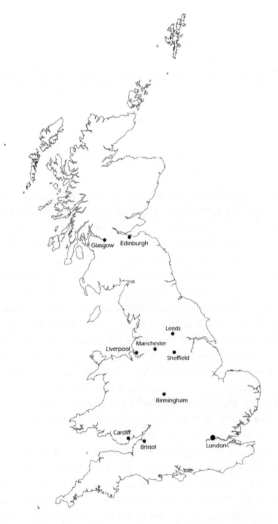

Figure 2.1 Major cities in early twentieth-century Britain

of population – which grew to over 400,000 in the later interwar years – and more with its economic and cultural significance as a major site of imperial trade, including famously the slave trade. Although it was not without some deep and highly visible social problems, the city's trading wealth furnished it with hospitals and numerous other philanthropic efforts in response.

Bristol's hospitals played an important role both within and beyond the city boundaries, providing medical education and specialist services for the South West of England. In this Bristol served as a regional capital, a key aspect of the 'hierarchical regionalism' Daniel Fox has suggested was characteristic of healthcare over the twentieth century.[3] Before surveying the city's hospitals, however, we should put them in their local context. In particular, we should locate them within the city's mixed economy of welfare and the characteristics of the city that forged that mix. Indeed, the diversity and plurality of welfare provision in Britain's past was especially evident in the case of Bristol. The absence of 'gas and water' socialism – with municipal control of utilities providing a bedrock – did not equate to a lack of provision in the city. Utilities, like other core services such as public transport, were provided by private companies.[4] Meanwhile, charitable provision was extensive, including schools, settlements and almshouses, as well as dispensaries and hospitals. Consequently, Bristol was a city associated with philanthropists well-known in their day, such as Edward Colston, George Muller, Mary Carpenter and Hannah Moore.[5] It might be expected that this left little space for public activity, and indeed this has been the charge of Alan DiGaentano.[6] Yet the city was also home to the first Board of Guardians in England when the Bristol Corporation of the Poor was founded in 1696.[7] From this early start, Bristol kept pace with the typical municipal developments of later centuries. Following wide-ranging sanitary reform in the mid-nineteenth century, municipal welfare activity underwent a notable expansion into the twentieth century.[8] Bristol's mixed economy of welfare therefore saw significant activity in all sectors.

This chapter will examine why the voluntary sector and wider mixed economies of healthcare, welfare and public services should be so well developed in Bristol. To do so, we will consider the social, economic and political factors at play in the city. Doing so allows to us ask what this meant for the hospitals operating in Bristol during the early twentieth century, which will be briefly surveyed. Embedding the wider picture in this local perspective is important if we are to understand what about the place and meaning of payment and philanthropy in the pre-NHS hospitals was due to the local factors and what was characteristic of British healthcare more widely.

Characteristics of the city

Economy and wealth

The foundation of Bristol's historic wealth, and consequent philanthropic dynamism, was trade. Its position as 'a bustling gateway of
empire trading' in the eighteenth century is well known.[9] However, a
number of historians have begun to bring Bristol's earlier trading history
out from the shadows of its Atlantic heyday.[10] The city's geographical
position afforded it earlier advantages in domestic trade as well, increasingly so as shipping, road and rail developments brought greater integration with the markets of England's South East and Midlands, and
then internationally.[11] Equally, the city's economic history since its
eighteenth-century heyday has also undergone some revision, with
focus moving away from early nineteenth-century failures in the private
management of the city docks and Bristol's subsequent usurpation by
Liverpool and Glasgow.[12] Amongst those offering a more positive
assessment have been Charles Harvey and Jon Press:

> Bristol has not been home to many giant corporations nor has any single
> industry ever dominated the local economy, yet what the region has
> lacked in terms of size and specialisation has been more than compen-
> sated for in terms of industrial diversity and economic flexibility. The
> economy of the Bristol region may not have grown as rapidly as many
> others in the nineteenth and twentieth centuries, but nor has it suffered
> the traumas of retrenchment that lately has afflicted so many British
> towns and cities.[13]

This trend whereby Bristol was economically well-suited to weather
national trends can be seen from unemployment and poor law statistics
up until the 1970s.[14]

The city's successful trading culture led to a sizeable and culturally
active middle-class elite.[15] When Charles Madge, co-founder of the
Mass Observation movement, surveyed patterns of household saving
in Bristol in 1940, he found 18.2 per cent to have weekly incomes above
£7.[16] This was notably more than the 12 per cent nationally with weekly
incomes over £5, according to the Ministry of Labour in 1938.[17] Meanwhile local surveys in both 1884 and 1937 concluded that, for the other
four-fifths of Bristolians, living standards were high and death rates low.
Figure 2.2 shows the 1937 income levels of the city's working-class
families, excluding the middle-class fifth of the population. 12.2 per

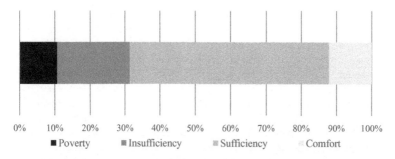

Figure 2.2 Working-class living standards in Bristol, 1937

cent were living in a state of 'comfort', defined as those with incomes at least 200 per cent higher than the BMA's harshly calculated minimum need. With an average gross income of 117s 6d per week, their lifestyle was described as 'very comfortable by the prevailing standard of the classes covered', allowing 'a margin for holidays, savings and luxuries'. A further 56.8 per cent were said to be living in a state of 'sufficiency', with incomes ranging between 50 per cent and 200 per cent above the minimum and an average gross income of 75s 10d per week. This was described as 'the ordinary standard of a Bristol working family' with 'some margin for saving or pleasure if they are frugal'. Another 20.8 per cent were said to live in a state of 'insufficiency', with an income above the minimum but less than 50 per cent above it, and an average gross income of 50s 2d per week. This was described as the 'scanty means' of those who 'whilst not in poverty, have a hard struggle, and whose lot is far from comfortable'. The final 10.7 per cent were those with incomes below the survey's calculated minimum needs, with an average gross income of 34s per week, and so deemed as 'in poverty'.[18] While not without poverty, therefore, Bristol was a wealthy city.

Health and housing
The 1884 survey had emphasised that 'With regard to health the inhabitants of Bristol are singularly favoured'.[19] This was said to be a recent development, with the situation rather different before slum clearances and sanitary reforms had taken effect:

> Then – not to speak of cellar dwellings and houses and rooms ill-built, out of repair, unventilated, with privies in sleeping and living rooms, and

over-crowding – there were private drains, cesspools, sewers, ash and refuse heaps – (sometimes one of these last at the house door or the end of every court, and left to be removed at pleasure); unmade roads ('not taken to' by the authorities) in fairly populous parts of the town; public manure heaps; privies emptying into open ditches; open sewers discharging putrid animal matter into the river, often in the freshes left to decompose upon the meads; water (often no *hard* water obtainable) deficient and tainted. But now there are 150 miles of sewerage, not such a thing as an open ditch, all ejects are trapped, a constant system of inspection, scavengering, limewashing, disinfecting is vigorously at work, and a water supply which, though here and there it may be inadequate, and is unfortunately retained in private hands, and is not therefore under the control of the public authorities, is pure and good.[20]

As sanitation was improved, death rates fell.[21] By 1883, Bristol had the lowest infant mortality rate (133 per 1,000 births) out of the twenty-eight large towns in England and was the only city with an overall death-rate below eighteen per 1,000.[22] In the early 1930s, a Ministry of Health report on the city noted that the death rate continued to be lower than the average for a county borough, despite recent epidemics of influenza and measles.[23] Beneath these low death rates, however, Bristol was home to notable health inequalities. This was evident from the geographical variation in mortality rates. In central areas it was 30 per cent higher than the city's interwar mean. In Westbury-on-Trym, which saw the lowest of the lower rates across the city's northern suburbs, it was 25 per cent below. There were exceptions, notably with a falling death rate from Congenital Debility and consistently lower infant and maternal mortality rates in the poor city centre. Hazlehurst attributes the latter to the movement in this period of the poorest families from central slums to new suburban corporation housing estates that were not as healthy as might have been expected.[24]

Even with new housing estates, the 1931 census reported greater 'housing pressure' in Bristol than any other part of Gloucestershire. Some 80.37 per cent of the city's occupied properties were home to a single family, while 16.18 per cent were home to two families and 3.45 per cent were home to three or more. Thirty-six per cent of families in Bristol shared their dwelling. The city-wide average was 1.25 families to each dwelling, with the rates for the nearby urban districts of Kingswood and Mangotsfield also high at 1.10 in both cases.[25] This reflected the wider concentration of regional population in Bristol. The city was consistently home to half of the population in the Gloucestershire area as it grew over the early twentieth century.[26]

What emerges from an examination of housing, health and the economy is a picture of significant social problems within an otherwise prosperous and healthy city. 'As a large, long-established city,' Martin Gorsky has suggested, 'Bristol can illustrate the concentration of needs which provided the demand for the voluntary sector and the emergence of the wealth which would finance the response to that demand.'[27] Moreover, the concentration of population brought visibility to Bristol's inequalities and social ills. In the words of one late-Victorian visitor to the city: 'I doubt if such striking contrasts between the two great divisions of the human race – the haves and the haves-nots – are presented anywhere else so vividly as in Bristol.'[28] Similarly, when in the mid-1870s volunteers from Clifton College arrived in St Agnes, a poor area just two miles from their public school, they found:

> Muck-heaps and farm-refuse, on which jerry-builders had set up rows of houses, which periodically got flooded, and suck up fever and death from chill for the poor folk who lodged therein. No lamps. Streets only wadeable through. A few public-houses of the worst sort surrounded a bit of open ground which was called 'the gardens', in which were tumble-down low huts of squatters in old time. These dwellers were the pick of the neighbourhood.[29]

Riots and strikes

If the visibility of poverty was a prompt for social action, so too was the level of agitation and disorder in the city.[30] Civil unrest has been a notable feature of Bristol's history and one with the power to undermine the local 'high-minded, well-ordered belief in progress'.[31] The response to riots over a new Bridge tax in 1793 led the poet Samuel Taylor Coleridge to claim that, if it was a Bristolian virtue to shoot unarmed civilians, 'I glory that I am an alien to your city.'[32] A different perspective was offered by one critical commentator on a weekend of political riots by 'Bristol mob-reformers' in 1831, when it was said 'the rioters were masters of the city'.[33] A similar sense of lawlessness was characterised during the 1980 St Paul's race riots by a police chief being heard to exclaim: 'Surely we should be advancing, not retreating?'[34]

Between these dramatic episodes, however, Bristol saw prolonged periods of calm, which were often out of step with the national mood, as had been the case when Bristol saw little of the chartist activity seen elsewhere.[35] Our chronological focus covers the end of a period of high tension in the city, which had taken hold in the 1880s, with notable radicalisation around industrial matters, unemployment and poverty.[36] Where the economic turbulence of earlier decades had been largely felt by the city's small firms with un-unionised workers, things were different by the end of the nineteenth century. Traditionally, Bristol's diversity was reflected in its series of small craft unions who saw their job as providing information to the public on matters relating to the local workers and poor.[37] Following a politicisation oriented firmly towards the Liberal Party in the 1870s, there was an 'upsurge of militancy' and union membership, which saw 'strike followed by strike in the city'.[38] This unrest continued into the interwar years, as strike action was taken by dockers, seamen, gasworkers, miners and transport workers.[39] Therefore the introduction of payment into the working-class experience of hospital treatment took place against a backdrop of social discord.

Following the First World War there were notable tensions around the situation of returning servicemen in three areas: public services, including the hospitals; public support, especially poor law relief; and unemployment alongside the continued employment of women. The position of ex-servicemen as patients in the Bristol Royal Infirmary was insecure, as seen when military patients were limited to 200 at any one time after a tense stand-off when 300 of them had refused to vacate their beds to make way for a venereal disease clinic in February 1919.[40] Two years later the public postwar donation benefit paid to ex-servicemen was ended in favour of poor law unemployment relief. The poor law guardians' offices were targeted in demonstrations, prompting an increase to the relief scales in September 1921. Meanwhile, ex-servicemen especially suffered in a climate of 'craft restrictions' where vocational opportunities were severely limited.[41] Discontent with female employment spilled over into a series of attacks on the city's trams in April 1920, after which women were no longer employed to work on them.[42] Although it had been suggested male workers might strike in solidarity with the female tram workers if dismissed, there appears to have been little appetite to put this into practice.[43] Across the interwar period female employment in the city in fact varied greatly. It peaked at 6,930 in December 1930, but from 1933 until the end of the decade it remained consistently low at between 1,500 and 2,000.[44]

The wider picture in the early 1920s was one of 'exceptional militancy', with protests and outbreaks of violence commonplace and allegations of brutality made against the police in 1921. However, strikes became something of a rarity after the demoralising resolution of the General Strike of 1926, in which 36,000 of Bristol's workers became involved.[45] The period of greatest militancy therefore came a decade before the period of greatest unemployment.

Electoral politics

Some explanation for this may be found in the co-ordination of the local labour movement, allowing for a rechanneling of efforts from protest to electoral politics. This was rather different from the late nineteenth century, when the city's labour and socialist movement was more of a social one, complete with its songbooks and summer picnics, as well as public lectures from the likes of William Morris and 'quiet talks by the way on intricacies of economics and sociology'.[46] Between the election of the city's first Labour councillors in 1887 and the outbreak of war in 1914, however, Duncan Tanner viewed Bristol's to have been one of the two 'most successful Labour organisations' in the country, the other being Leicester. He attributed this to the strength, especially in the poorer east of the city, of the 600-strong Independent Labour Party (ILP).[47] Thereafter the merger of the Trades Council with the Labour Party in 1919 is also significant, as is the 1921 foundation of the Bristol Unemployed Association, which had established a close working relationship with the Trades Council and links with Labour by the end of the decade.[48] When the local parliamentary breakthrough came in 1923, Labour won the Bristol East and North seats, also taking Bristol South in 1929.[49] Since 1945 Labour has usually held the majority of Bristol seats.

Figure 2.3 shows both the success of Labour in Westminster elections since 1945 and the earlier dominance of the Liberals, stretching from the 1830s to the 1920s. In local politics, however, the situation was very different. It was in fact the Tories and then Conservatives that had control of the city council from 1812 until 1904, suggesting there was little difference between the merchant oligarchy before the 1835 Municipal Corporations Act and the reformed chamber thereafter.[50] An

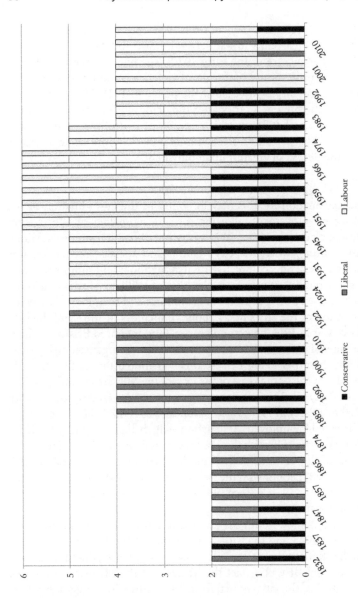

Figure 2.3 Party distribution of MPs in Bristol since 1832

outright Liberal majority in 1904 was denied by Labour's five council-lors, while Conservative dominance of the Aldermanic bench contin-ued. Although 1906 saw the Liberals increase their representation to hold three of the city's four seats in its landslide general election victory, the same year also saw them lose their position as the largest party on the council for another century.[51] By 1925 Labour had increased its number of councillors from five to eighteen out of the sixty-nine total, and again to thirty-two in 1930. These successes and the parallel Liberal struggles prompted the formation of an 'anti-socialist' alliance, with Labour facing the Citizen Party in local elections between 1926 and 1973. This arrangement not only held off a Labour majority for a decade but also ensured clear control of the council until 1945. Between 1945 and 2002, however, no period without a Labour majority lasted more than three years.[52]

As 'a distinctly local reaction to the rise of the Labour Party', the Citizen Party was able to position itself as a localist rejection of the nationalising agenda of Labour when in government at Westminster.[53] Their pamphlets and cartoons at the time of the 1947 local elections portray the local party simply doing the bidding of a failing central government.[54] Despite this, we should also bear in mind that the city had, in W.H. Ayles, leader of the Bristol ILP, a champion of 'decentral-ised municipal Socialism', a philosophy put forward in his 1921 *What a Socialist Town Council Should Be*.[55] It would not be correct, however, to solely explain the rise of municipalism in Bristol by the growth of the Labour Party as a political force. This was a trend becoming established in parallel to the foundation of Labour organisations in the city, as the Liberals responded to the city's radical tradition.[56] Indeed, the remit of the council had expanded from its ten committees in 1875, increasing to twenty-three by 1915.[57] This expansion asserted the place of public provision as an essential element of an established and diverse mixed economy in the city's welfare and public services, to which we now turn.

The mixed economy of welfare

Poor law
The earliest pillar of Bristol's mixed economy of welfare was the poor law. As early as 1696 the city's eighteen parishes and the ward of castle

precincts collaborated to bring about the Bristol Corporation of the Poor, the first Board of Guardians in England, with the city's old mint serving as both administrative centre and workhouse. However, this did not equate to a high level of service. By 1831, there were 600 inmates in this crowded workhouse, with ten beds for fifty-eight girls and seventeen for seventy-eight boys.[58] Following the 1834 Poor Law Amendment Act, the Bristol Corporation Union was joined by another two. These were the Clifton Union, covering the Gloucestershire suburbs to the north, and the Bedminster Union, serving the Somerset suburbs to the south.[59] In 1844, the Clifton Union's Pennywell Road workhouse was visited by an Assistant Poor Law Commissioner, who reported both workhouse and inmates to be 'filthy and wretched', with 'men, women and children being indiscriminately herded together'.[60] Associations with poverty and high mortality rates saw the name changed to Barton Regis in 1877, distinguishing it from the wealthy parish and desirable health resort of Clifton.[61]

The three unions were amalgamated in 1898, following the 1894 Local Government Act. Their amalgamation allowed for greater 'moral classification', including separating out the 'Deserving Aged'. By this time the new union had 2,357 inmates spread across four workhouses (Stapleton, Eastville, Bedminster and St Peter's Hospital), and another (Southmead) was built in 1902. The early twentieth century did not only see the expansion of workhouses, but also new schemes. For example, in 1922 the Guardians began putting men receiving Unemployment Relief to work cultivating their land in Downend. The 1920s also saw the increasing use of emigration as a welfare policy in Bristol, most notably to Canada and Australia.[62]

Philanthropy

The poor law was one of the two pillars of Victorian welfare. The other was philanthropy. The historic prominence of philanthropic associations in Bristol was acknowledged in a Ministry of Health report on the city in the 1930s:

> The religious enthusiasm evoked by Whitfield and Wesley still to some extent remains ... Bristol is well served with charities and voluntary organisations, many of which are ecclesiastical in origin, and the City is especially fortunate in possessing a comparatively large number of

wealthy citizens who are at the same time generous benefactors where municipal interests are concerned.[63]

Foremost amongst these benefactors were the tobacco-magnate Wills family, who funded the landmark university buildings as well as supplying a string of presidents for and substantial donations to the city's hospitals. Philanthropic work and municipal governance alike had a proud pedigree amongst the city's merchants, reaching back to Edward Colston.[64] Bristol as an international city was reflected in the campaigning activities of the Indian social reformer Rajah Rammohan Roy in the early nineteenth century, and the orphanages founded by George Muller, son of a Russian exciseman, later in the century.[65] At the same time, these philanthropic activities provided social networks within which women were able to interact not only with each other but also with new areas of public life, such as politics. Best remembered is Mary Carpenter, for her Reformatory and Industrial Schools from the 1830s. However, the late nineteenth century saw these associations also provide a platform for more radical campaigns, such as Frances Power Cobbe's for women's property rights.[66]

Philanthropy was also a common activity of the city's less prestigious, middle-class citizens.[67] Over the 1870s and 1880s, for example, the St Agnes Workmen's Club developed out of the Clifton College school mission-rooms. By the 1890s the mission had turned its 'attention to the wants of the boys in the neighbourhood', running summer camps and establishing a Boys' Club. This provided activities including football, cricket, gymnastics and swimming, all intended to offer 'the help and discipline of life that they needed'. Following which a Girls' Club was started, running camps and classes in embroidery. The mission was understood to provide 'the boys of Bristol' with 'an education' through 'contact with the life of a Public School', whereby they 'learnt something of the public spirit, the *spirit de corps* so essential to a true life'. Meanwhile, it showed 'the boys of the School ... quite another side of life'.[68]

Martin Gorsky has noted in his study of charity in nineteenth-century Bristol that:

> societies and subscriber institutions provided a means of addressing social problems which neither market nor state could tackle, the former because the purchase of social insurance, good education and health care was beyond the means of many, and the latter because the broad range

of consensus for social spending obtained only for the extremes of disadvantage: lunacy, the destitute, the aged and infirm.[69]

Not only did the voluntary sector in the nineteenth century operate in a space the public and private sectors were incapable of filling, but it also made a different contribution to the social fabric of the city. Victorian philanthropy in Bristol was, as Gorsky has noted, 'a relation between have and have-not', and this cannot be said in the same way of the era's municipal or commercial solutions to social problems.[70] However, the city's historians have not universally taken such a positive view of philanthropy. Mary Fissell emphasised the 'factionalized nature of charity and relief in the city', describing charitable acts in eighteenth-century Bristol as both an 'expression of civic unity' and an 'articulation of social difference'.[71] Helen Meller's work on leisure examined how Bristol's middle-class elite embarked on a Victorian mission to bring about a unifying culture of 'social citizenship' in the city. While she was less critical of the mission itself, she concluded that the vision remained ultimately unrealised.[72] While philanthropy did not bring about social harmony or unity in Bristol, it was undoubtedly a major feature of the social life of the city.

Municipal activity

Although philanthropic activity was extensive in the city, it would be wrong to see it as a substitute for public provision. Municipal interventionism, in both economic and social fields, was evident in Bristol from the early to mid-nineteenth century. Following the 1831 riots there were calls for policing reform, and following legislation the city established a public constabulary in 1836.[73] When an outbreak of cholera claimed 445 lives in 1849, the response was to establish the corporation's sanitary committee in 1851.[74] This signalled the adoption of the permissive 1848 Public Health Act, which included responsibility for the maintenance of streets and lighting alongside the introduction of a modern drainage system, designed to intercept sewage and prevent it from flowing into the harbour. It was a major function of the council, coming by the 1870s to account for more than half of its expenditure.[75] However, this action did not entirely put an end to the problem, simply transporting the sewage to the banks of the River Avon, with inaction continuing to prevent a more comprehensive project for decades thereafter.[76]

Meanwhile, there were developments continuing in other areas of public provision. The public School Board took over the work of religious groups running fee-paying schools and Clifton College's ragged school, working 'among neglected boys', which had reached over 18,000 pupils.[77] There were also public developments in utilities. Amongst the late nineteenth-century municipal committees set up was the electricity committee, in 1884, with one of England's earliest public power stations by 1893.[78] However, public control of such provision was limited, allowing an 1891 Fabian pamphlet to critique:

> Bristol is in many respects the most backward of English municipalities. Most important towns in England own their own waterworks: Bristol leaves this vital public service in the hands of a monopolist company earning a dividend of eight and a half per cent. Two-thirds of the gas consumers in the United Kingdom are supplied by municipal enterprise: Bristol depends for light on a company earning ten per cent. More than a quarter of the tramways in this country are owned by public authorities: Bristol allows private adventurers to earn five per cent. by running cars through the public streets. Birmingham, Manchester, Bradford and many other places keep all three of these public services under public control for public profit. Bristol enjoys the bad pre-eminence of being the largest provincial municipality which allows all three to remain in private hands for private advantage.[79]

Housing might also have been added to this list, as the critique of the Council for not implementing the 1890 Housing of the Working Classes Act was heard from those first Labour councillors.[80]

Private enterprise

If action was slower than many wanted from local government, there was significant activity from other sectors, including private enterprise, as can be seen from the case of private asylums. Dr Edward Long Fox opened the first at Cleve Hill in 1794, two years before the more famous York Retreat, before moving to Brislington House a decade later. As such, this private asylum for the treatment of an elite clientele was one of the first purpose-built institutions for the care of the insane in Britain.[81] At the same time there were developments in the commercial provision of public services, such as the private Bristol Gas Light Company's introduction of gas street lights to the city within a decade of London setting the precedent in 1810.[82] Meanwhile, the 1846 establishment of the private Water Works Company was a direct response to the poor water supply, and was consciously seen as part of the public health reforms of the city; although it was a source of contention and there were calls for municipalisation until improvements in the 1870s.[83] Equally, the interwar years have been remembered as the 'heyday' of the city's private transport system, with both trams, not yet affected by the wartime bombing of 1941, and the Bristol Tramways' taxi service operating in the city, until the latter was made uneconomical by the growth of car ownership in 1932.[84] This private provision of public services continued through the early twentieth century until, just like the voluntary hospitals, they were caught up in the sweeping nationalisations of the postwar Labour government.

The changing mix of public and private can also be seen in the field of general practice. The 1911 National Insurance Act had introduced the panel system, whereby compulsory insurance for workers in selected industries would provide access to a doctor when taken ill. This system expanded over the interwar period, when it came to cover the majority of the adult population, alongside a parallel growth in the still more profitable private practice.[85] In the case of Bristol, we should note the prominence of Clifton as a location for general practice surgeries. In this one area were the surgeries of all the voluntary hospitals' consultants and a significant minority of the GPs in the whole city. However, as table 2.1 shows, this concentration was actually in decline over the interwar years. Over the 1920s there was an increase in the number of GP surgeries in Clifton before nearly half this growth was reversed in the following decade. Across the city as a whole, there was a growth of one-fifth in the first decade, then a marginal increase in the second. There was a lessening of the concentration of the city's general

Table 2.1 General practice surgeries in Bristol, 1919–39

	Bristol	Clifton	(%)	Bedminster	(%)
1919	226	88	38.9	12	5.3
1930	274	102	37.2	19	6.9
1939	280	93	33.2	33	11.8

Source: Wright's and Kelly's Directories for Bristol.

practitioners in this one elite area, and an expansion in other areas. These included the city's suburbs in the north (such as Westbury-on-Trym) and the south (including Knowle), but was most prominent in working-class areas such as Bedminster. This was an area on the south of the river, home to much of the industry and many of the labourers associated with the city docks, and table 2.1 shows general practice growing in this part of Bristol, especially in the 1930s as the local economy was recovering.[86]

Health and welfare

Municipal provision in the wider field of health also expanded in this period. An interventionist approach might be expected under Labour, yet they did not chair the Health Committee until the end of the 1930s. For almost the entire interwar period the Chairman was Herbert John Maggs, a notable figure in the local Liberal Party. Maggs served as a St George and Central ward councilor from 1906, alderman from 1927 and mayor in 1932. In the early 1930s, a Ministry of Health report noted that he 'has had an almost unbroken connection with the Health Committee since 1906 and he has been its Chairman for the last 10 years.'[87] Given the wide-ranging remit of the Health Committee, it allows us to reconsider the supposed Conservative domination of the Citizen Party in this area.

The eagerness for municipal expansion in this field can be seen from the case of nourishment grants. For some time these provisions, usually of milk, had been part of tubercular care in the city. The Health Committee unquestioningly adhered to the Tuberculosis Officer's recommendations on who should receive them, and as a preventive measure this came to include many poor expectant and nursing mothers and infants.[88] This raised a complaint from the Town Clerk, who said this fell beyond the powers granted by Local Government Board Regulations, declaring himself to be 'of the opinion that the Corporation cannot legally make any payment in respect of food or nourishment to mothers or children.'[89] The disagreement was resolved the following year when the 1918 Maternity and Child Welfare Act granted local authorities exactly this power.[90] The number of nourishment grants increased following the Act and again in the late 1920s, when an investigation into the increase found six out of seven applicants were unemployed.[91] By the mid-1930s Bristol's annual spend of around £3,000 on milk grants was similar to those Dr Dorothy Taylor's Ministry of Health study found in Reading, Chelmsford and Shoreditch, significantly less than Manchester, and notably greater than Gloucester, Leicester, Northampton, Woolwich or Barking.[92] This is in line with overall spending on maternity and child welfare, which was middling nationally but behind only its wealthy neighbour of Bath in the South West.[93] Once again, activity in this area was not restricted to one sector. In fact, the majority of municipal spending over the interwar years went on contracts for the voluntary Bristol Infant Welfare Association to provide mother and infant clinics across the city.[94]

Universalism

Bristol's history is then one of local readiness to take on new powers, sometimes even pre-empting their legal empowerment, and then to extend activities in various fields of social welfare. This was also evident ahead of the 1929 Local Government Act that nominally ended the poor law. The response from the Board of Guardians to the high rate of unemployment and hardship in the 1920s was often to ignore 'the restrictive means test applied to indoor and outdoor relief' in an effort 'to ease suffering'. It was a grassroots administrative rejection of the Victorian notion of less eligibility and the creed of utilitarianism, moving instead 'towards the incipient beginnings of universal and equitable relief which was to become a central tenet of the Welfare State.'[95]

This universalism was symptomatic of a new age, one distinctly different from that of the poor law and Victorian philanthropy. The effect of this shift on charitable activity was certainly a concern of the Bristol Charity Organization Society (COS), who feared the 1906 Liberal Government's reforms would make 'Socialism … a real factor in the life of the community.'[96] The impact of local and national welfare initiatives was seen in a dramatic fall of more than two-thirds in applications to the Bristol COS (or Civic League as it was renamed): from 1,234 in 1907 to only 378 in 1927.[97] This trend was reversed over the 1930s, with the number of applicants steadily rising to over 2,000 in 1940.[98] The continued increase during economic recovery can be explained by a move away from grants and loans in favour of services 'not concerned with the actual giving of money.'[99] The League was better placed to meet local needs by providing advice on landlords and moneylenders as well as public and charitable sources of support. This was aided by opening offices in the new housing estates in Knowle West and Southmead, which provided over half the League's cases by the 1940s.[100] The work of the League in these new districts could sometimes hark back to its COS origins, such as the establishment of a 'thrift club' in Knowle West 'to defeat the present system of purchasing everything possible on credit'.[101] The early 1940s, however, saw their focus settle on the areas that would be left for the voluntary sector in the age of the postwar welfare state. This included a register of homeless people and work on old people's welfare, but most notably a wartime enquiry bureau and the longer-lasting 'Citizen's Friend' scheme with its 'Poor Man's Lawyer Service'.[102]

Welfare across the mixed economy

The charge DiGaetano has levelled at Bristol is that only municipal developments in the twentieth century rescued the city from a failed private/voluntary model of public services.[103] This description does not fit a history of early interventions, even if followed up less extensively than elsewhere, and a genuinely dynamic mixed economy across many areas, including medical and social welfare. The areas where municipal activity was limited in the nineteenth century were those same areas where commercial and philanthropic activity was considerable. Moreover, this mix continued in the twentieth century as provision from all sides expanded. It was not until after the Second World War, as Martin Gorsky has noted, specifically citing Bristol's hospitals, 'that the role of charity in core services came to be considered inappropriate'.[104] At least until this time, the voluntary sector was part of the diverse and pluralistic tapestry of service providers that made up the city's evolving mixed economy of welfare.

Voluntary hospitals

Within this mixed economy we find the city's hospitals.[105] While the voluntary hospitals were leading charitable institutions in their own right, they were also deeply embedded within local networks of care. By the 1930s, the social work functions of the almoners, principally securing financial support and after-care arrangements for patients, had brought the hospitals into closer partnership with a wide range of

local organisations, ranging from the Rotary Club to the university settlements and the local *Times and Mirror* Relief Fund.[106] In some cases
almoners made arrangements with voluntary bodies focused on health,
including the hospital contributory schemes, district nurses, ambulance corps and various local funds for surgical appliances, while others
supported specific groups, such as crippled children, military families
or those with disabilities. In other cases they collaborated with religious
organisations, ranging from the Bristol Diocesan Moral Welfare Association and the Waifs and Strays Society to the Catholic Women's
League. The hospitals worked with a host of public bodies, including
the Unemployment Assistance Board and a variety of municipal committees including on education, health and housing, as well as institutions already bringing together public and voluntary welfare providers,
such as Infant Welfare Centres. The voluntary hospitals had long-
standing arrangements with partners as varied as central government
committees and a regular 'anonymous donor for help with Insulin'.[107]
Firmly entrenched as hubs at the centre of these local networks of care,
and at the intersection of the mixed economy of welfare, were the hospitals themselves (see Figure 2.4).

General hospitals

'An Infirmary at Bristol for the benefit of the poor sick', one of the first
outside London,[108] took its first patients in December 1737 – seventeen
men and seventeen women.[109] Its foundation was in line with the 'liberal
ethos, in which Christianity and commerce neatly joined', and 'the city's
merchant elite' were the base from which the institution was established; and the city's deputy Controller of Customs, John Elbridge,
conceived of the idea and became the Bristol Royal Infirmary's (BRI)
first treasurer.[110] This tie with the city's wealthy business community
remained strong into the interwar period, with the 'plutocratic benevo-
lence' of the industrialist Wills family, which provided both numerous
presidents and significant financial donations to the BRI and other
voluntary hospitals in the city.[111] This was a notable enough feature for
it to be joked in 1934 that the city had been relying on the old adage:
'Where there's a Wills, there's a way'.[112] Certainly the BRI was an institution for which charitable donations large and small continued to be
important – although the interwar years saw this decline from a majority to under one-third of ordinary income.[113] Still, the BRI was notably

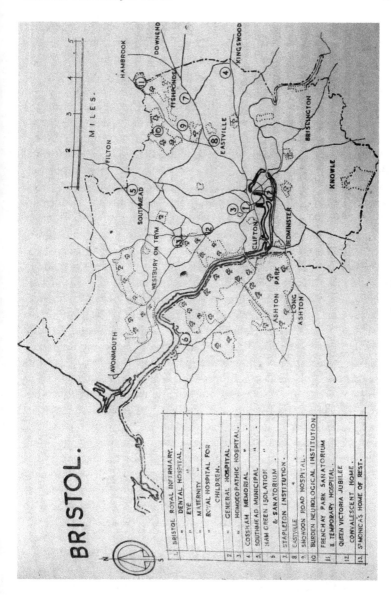

Figure 2.4 Hospitals in Bristol in the 1940s

an institution established and governed by the city's elite long before it officially became the Bristol *Royal* Infirmary. The divisions within this elite, between Whigs and Tories and between Church and Dissent, were evident in late 1770s elections of the Infirmary's governors, which were said to have a 'strong political flavour'.[114]

Political divisions in the city added to the case for the founding of a second general hospital, opened in 1831 on the waterfront on the industrial south of the river.[115] This industrial setting meant that, along-side the patronage of the Wills family, the Bristol General Hospital (BGH) benefited from workpeople's donations at a rate proportion-ately three times higher than the BRI.[116] Beyond concerns one hospital could not meet existing demand, there was also desire for a politically different kind of institution.[117] The city's two sitting Whig members of parliament were heavily associated with the new hospital, as was George Thomas of the influential local family of Liberal Quakers.[118] The new hospital was founded amidst the city's Reform riots, and 'it was said that patients going to the Infirmary would receive a sovereign remedy, but those at the Hospital a radical cure'.[119] These differences were overcome when, in a gradual process between 1939 and 1942, the former's 425 beds and the latter's 269 were merged to form the Bristol Royal Hospital. Between them and then combined, they provided a major regional centre. Although nearly three-quarters of BRI patients were from Bristol, notable numbers came from further afield – one in ten patients was from Somerset and slightly more from Gloucester-shire.[120] The position of Bristol and specifically the BRI as the regional centre was reinforced when it became the site for the consolidated Bristol Medical and Surgical School, making the institution the South West hub for specialist services and training.[121] By the Second World War 45.5 per cent of its beds were set aside for specialist treatments, with maternity, ear, nose and throat (ENT), orthopaedic and gynaeco-logical services prominent. While the General Hospital had a focus on general and surgical provision, they offered specialisms such as radio-therapy not available at the BRI.[122] A demonstration of this regional capital status had already been seen in the First World War, when the BRI's new King Edward VII Memorial Wing had served as the poorly reimbursed headquarters for the Southern General No. 2 under the direction of the War Office.[123]

Specialist hospitals

Bristol's role as a regional specialist hub was not restricted to services in the general hospitals. An 'Institution for the cure of Diseases of the Eye among the Poor' was established in Bristol in 1810, only five years after the first at the London Moorfields. This was an early example of a major nineteenth-century wave of hospitals founded not by charitable benefactors but by medical men.[124] Although the medical man in question, Surgeon Oculist William Henry Goldwyer, was aided by the patronage of the Duke of Gloucester and the involvement of the Freemasons.[125] In 1939 the Eye Hospital's eighty-four beds were being utilised primarily by patients from the city, but one in ten were from Gloucestershire and one in five from Somerset with most of the others from South Wales.[126]

Another specialist institution founded later in the nineteenth century was the Home for Crippled Children. From 1875 this served as a hospital for children (boys from six months until aged seven, girls ten), employing 'sun treatments' to treat infantile paralysis, talipes and spinal curvature or disease, and sometimes from rickets. These patients were usually sponsored by their local municipal health committee.[127] The Bristol hospital was closed in 1930, with most of the institution's management committee and patients moved seven miles south to Winford in Somerset.[128] Most of the patients at the Winford Orthopaedic Hospital (also known as the 'Bristol Crippled Children's Open Air Hospital') suffered from rheumatic heart disease, many of whom were council-funded non-pulmonary tubercular patients.[129]

Also founded in the late nineteenth century was the Children's Hospital, beginning in 1857 as a dispensary and settling in 1885 at the site it would occupy for over a century.[130] The 'objects of the institution', unchanged for most of that time, were threefold:

1. – To provide for the reception, maintenance, and medical and surgical treatment of Children under thirteen years of age, in a suitable building, cheerfully and salubriously placed; to furnish with advice and medicine those who cannot or need not be admitted into the Hospital; and also to receive Women suffering from disease peculiar to their sex.

2. – To promote the advancement of medical science with reference to the diseases of Women and Children, and to provide for the instruction of Students in these essential departments of medical knowledge.

3. – To diffuse among all classes of the community, and particularly among the poor, a better acquaintance with the management of Infants and Children during health and sickness; and to assist in the education and training of Women in the special duties of Children's Nurses.[131]

Nearly half of its 109 beds were for general medical cases, while it also provided a range of specialisms, including ENT and gynaecology.[132] Meanwhile, services for children over women were kept as the sole work of the hospital when war damage reduced it to only fifty-eight beds for inpatients.[133]

One notable figure in the history of the Children's Hospital was Eliza Walker Dunbar, appointed house surgeon in 1873 as the first female doctor in any of the city's hospitals. However, the response to the controversial appointment of a woman was a walk-out by the existing honorary staff. Despite the support of the governors, she soon resigned her post.[134] During this time she engaged with the city's notable network of women campaigners and philanthropists, including Miss Read. Bringing together the money of one and the professional training of the other, the Read Dispensary for Women and Children opened in 1874.[135] It relocated and reopened in 1896 as a hospital, and again in 1931 to sit alongside the city's elite private practices in the suburb of Clifton.[136] Following demand, the hospital shifted the focus of its thirty-two beds from general women's services to maternity during the 1930s. The institution's story is one of mission drift, from dispensary for the city's working classes to elite hospital primarily for paying patients.[137]

This was one of a number of maternity hospitals in the city. The Bristol Lying-In Institution, founded in 1865, had its origins in the earlier 'Bristol Pentientiary', designed to rehabilitate fallen women.[138] The new institution was still overtly moralistic, as emphasised in a letter published in the local *Western Daily Press* in 1886 encouraging donations:

Its object is the immediate shelter of young girls who have gone astray, and as such it is indispensable to the success of other branches of rescue work. Many who have been restored to a life of respectability and happiness acknowledge their indebtedness to the Christian influence exercised over them by ladies interested in the institution, and especially the excellent matron, who seldom fails to win the love and gratitude of those who have been for any length of time under her care.[139]

The early twentieth century, however, saw this change. After the First World War, as at the Salvation Army's Mount Hope maternity home, married women became the focus, while smaller institutions took over working with unmarried mothers.[140] Meanwhile growing demand for hospital births put pressure on the small Brunswick Maternity Hospital, which entered into a new arrangement with the local health committee in the 1920s. Using its new powers under the Maternity and Child Welfare Act of 1918 and backed by the Ministry of Health, they bought the property and rented it back to the hospital governors.[141] However, by the early 1930s, they decided to close the old Brunswick hospital, as maternity patients were increasingly being admitted to newer facilities.[142] Many of these were new wards at the BRI, which could claim that one-fifth of all Bristol births took place in their wards. The response of the Maternity Hospital was to complain of their 'reduced numbers' as a consequence and, in 1932, to poach the BRI's Matron. It was a rivalry that did not stand in the way of the fifty-bed Maternity Hospital amalgamating with the Bristol Royal Hospital in 1946.[143]

The picture across the city's maternity and other voluntary hospitals was one of financial difficulties and closures amidst an expansion of services. For instance, at the Children's Hospital, even as subscriptions declined, other forms of charitable income increased from around one-third of all ordinary income to nearly half over the interwar years.[144] The Wills family spent £13,000 on a new Homeopathic Hospital which opened in 1925, marking the death of Captain Bruce Melville Wills in France in 1915.[145] Developing the work of a nineteenth-century dispensary, it complemented the continuing operation of three dispensaries – two in the working-class areas of St Paul's and Bedminster, with another in nearby Weston-Super-Mare.[146] The significance of the Homeopathic Hospital is less the service its seventy-nine beds provided and more the demonstration that wealthy benefactors were still capable of founding voluntary hospitals in the city, even in the financially challenging days of the early 1920s.

Another similar demonstration was offered by the establishment of the Cossham Memorial Hospital in 1907. This was 'a general hospital for the treatment and relief of sick and injured persons of both sexes' established from the legacy of the Colliery owner, Liberal MP for Bristol East and two-time Mayor of Bath, Handel Cossham.[147] He had declared it his 'earnest wish that I may be hereafter remembered by the sick and suffering as a friend who in death as in life has felt it his duty to try and lessen human suffering and increase human happiness.'[148] With its 100 beds catering for local patients to the east of the city, it was described in the 1930s as being 'the largest casualty outpost in the City of Bristol'.[149] The hospital's 'Subscribers' were said to be 'lamentably small', 'only about one-fourth of what it should be'.[150] Meanwhile it established an early workers' governors committee: 'Without the help of these friends', the 1936 report said, 'the doors of many hospitals would have been closed or thrown back on the state'.[151] It serves, there-fore, as just one of the examples of voluntary sector expansion in the early twentieth century, alongside the city's public hospitals.

Public hospitals

Poor law infirmaries

Poor Law infirmaries have sometimes been seen as the nucleus of a public hospital service.[152] In Bristol this meant the sick wards of the workhouses (rebranded as public assistance institutions following the 1929 Local Government Act) at Stapleton and Eastville. A Ministry of Health survey in the early 1930s judged that Stapleton was essentially a public asylum, with fewer than one in five of its 796 patients not certi-fied.[153] Meanwhile, a great many of its patients were 'aged and infirm persons, who are mostly bedridden'.[154] Those in the 'sick' wards at East-ville were primarily treated for diseases of the skin and the respiratory and circulatory systems, for influenza and for senile decay.[155] As at Sta-pleton, however, over four-fifths of inmates were not medical cases. With an average age of sixty-eight for men and seventy-nine for women, half the bedridden inmates were suffering from chronic diseases, such as rheumatoid arthritis; the other half were 'bedridden purely on account of age' in 1930.[156] The Public Assistance Committee's response was the new Snowdon Road Hospital, which had expanded by 1943 to 478 patients, roughly one-fifth of whom were tubercular patients and most of the rest chronic sick cases.[157]

By the 1930s the largest hospital in the city was Southmead, one of the first poor law institutions to be purpose-built as a medical facility, completed just in time to be brought into the war effort until 1920.[158] A decade later, on 1 April 1930, Southmead was appropriated under the

1929 Local Government Act. As such, instead of passing from the poor law guardians to the Public Assistance Committee, as was the case with Stapleton and Eastville, it was transferred to the Health Committee 'to ensure that those persons who will receive from the Council by reason of their poor circumstances assistance in the form of hospital treatment shall do so in the same hospitals and under the same conditions as the rest of the citizens'.[159] Once again, Bristol had pre-empted this progressive change locally. Rather than catering only for paupers, the city's Medical Officer of Health told the voluntary hospitals that 'Some time ago the Board of Guardians opened the doors of Southmead for the treatment of sick persons of all classes'. Before appropriation 'roughly one half were not pauper patients', and the development of a general hospital for the whole community could therefore take place 'without dislocation'. The change was not designed to alter the hospital services on offer in the city, but rather to 'remove the stigma of pauperism'.[160] This goal was aided by a new maternity specialism, developed in partnership with the university, and increasing maternity admissions were heralded as a sign of success.[161] By 1943, the local press was reporting 2,600 yearly births at Southmead.[162]

Infectious disease sanatoria

Besides poor law infirmaries, public hospitals in the city were focused on infectious diseases. Following temporary arrangements, such as the use of the Port Sanitary Committee's 'Hospital Ship', persistent outbreaks of diphtheria prompted the establishment of two institutions.[163] One thirty-five bed isolation hospital was set up in the south of the city at Novers Hill, primarily treating smallpox and occasionally scarlet fever patients.[164] This was followed in 1899 by a much larger infectious disease hospital at Ham Green, on a site of ninety-nine acres with including a mansion and two farms, five miles from Bristol.[165] The initial focus at Ham Green was on diphtheria and smallpox, although temporary accommodation for tubercular cases gradually became more central.[166] By the 1930s it was a major centre for the treatment of infectious diseases, conducting medical research and developing new treatments for pulmonary tuberculosis, bronchitis and artificial pneumothorax.[167] While the medical work of Ham Green expanded, Novers Hill was transferred to the Education Committee in 1934 to become an open air school.[168] This was accompanied by a new 100-bed sanatorium and open air school for thirty children in a converted eighteenth-century Mansion House at Frenchay Park, to the north east of the city.[169] When 133 were hospitalised in a 1941 outbreak of measles, they were sent to another new public institution, Charterhouse Hospital, sixteen miles to the south of Bristol on the Mendip Hills.[170]

This period of expansion, with numerous new institutions established, had its limits. Bristol's spending on infectious disease in fact declined during the interwar years.[171] Southmead was appropriated and its clinical standards raised, yet its range of services remained far more focused on chronic and tubercular patients than the voluntary hospitals it sought to imitate. Meanwhile, other public assistance institutions were little changed since their days as workhouse infirmaries. The voluntary hospitals therefore remained the core of acute and specialist hospital provision in Bristol.

Conclusion

In Bristol's hospitals we therefore see reflected a number of defining characteristics of the city. The trading wealth and business connection that had founded the hospitals continued to provide leadership and financial support for expansion in the early twentieth century. This ensured both that Bristol served as the regional medical capital (discussed further in chapter 4) and that there were new institutions and services that needed financing, with one means of doing so being the introduction of patient payments. The city's early provincial appointment of almoners to set up payment schemes is in line with its eager adoption of some new health and welfare policies, even pre-empting empowerment from central government in some cases, while the slow establishment of the hospital contributory scheme movement (to which we will return in the next chapter) was more in keeping with the much-criticised reticence over collectivist approaches in other cases of welfare and public service provision. The pattern of expansion in health and welfare during the early twentieth century demonstrated that dual expansion was seen in public and voluntary sectors, rather than one crowding out or replacing the other. This trend of the two developing in concert, on increasingly common ground, is something seen in relation to the design and implementation of patient payment schemes. In many respects, therefore, we see the introduction of patient payment reflecting the defining characteristic of the city's mixed economies of health and welfare.

The economic, political and social life of the city during the early twentieth century does not only give us the framework for the arrival of payment in the hospitals, but also some insight into context within which it was experienced and understood at the time. Bristol was a wealthy city, but it was also one with significant social problems. These were exacerbated by the unemployment and economic turbulence that followed the First World War, which saw disputes, strikes and riots commonplace in what was, like many others, a febrile city. The rise of Labour as an electoral outlet for dissatisfaction rechannelled some of the tension in the city over the interwar years, but at the time when patient payments were being introduced there were protests over unemployment and retrenchment. While there is little evidence of resentment at being asked to contribute financially to the hospitals, as there was over changes to the benefits granted to ex-servicemen, it would be wrong to entirely separate the new financial dimension to hospital treatment from this wider context. Resented or not, the introduction of patient payments and the later admission of private patients to the voluntary hospitals did raise questions over their charitable nature. Philanthropy was not displaced, although it did undergo something of an identity crisis.

Notes

1 Nuffield Provincial Hospitals Trust, *The Hospital Surveys: The Domesday Book of Hospital Services* (Oxford: Oxford University Press, 1946), p. 4.
2 For British historic population figures, see the 'Visions of Britain' online resource at www.visionofbritain.org.uk, accessed 25 April 2016.
3 See Daniel M. Fox, *Health Policies, Health Politics: The British and American Experience, 1911–1965* (Princeton: Princeton University Press, 1986).
4 Harold Nabb, *The Bristol Gas Industry 1815–1949* (Bristol: Bristol Branch of the Historical Association, 1987); David Large, *The Municipal Government of Bristol, 1851–1901* (Bristol: Bristol Record Society, 1999); David Harrison, 'Safety, Speed, Comfort and Cheapness: Travel by Road, Rail and Water' in David Harrison (ed.) *Bristol between the Wars: A City and Its People 1919–1939* (Bristol: Redcliffe Press, 1984), pp. 45–55.
5 On the range of philanthropic activity, see Helen Meller, *Leisure and the Changing City, 1870–1914* (London: Routledge and Kegan Paul, 1976)

and Martin Gorsky, *Patterns of Philanthropy: Charity and Society in Nine-teenth-Century Bristol* (Woodbridge: Boydell & Brewer Ltd, 1999).

6 Alan DiGaetano, 'The Birth of Modern Urban Governance: A Compari-son of Political Modernization in Boston, Massachusetts, and Bristol, England, 1800–1870', *Journal of Urban History*, 35:2 (2009), 259–87.

7 Moira Martin, 'Managing the Poor: The Administration of Poor Relief in Bristol in the Nineteenth and Twentieth Centuries' in Madge Dresser and Philip Ollerenshaw (eds), *The Making of Modern Bristol* (Bristol: Redcliffe Press, 1996), pp. 157–8.

8 Gorsky, *Patterns of Philanthropy*, pp. 222–5; Large, *Municipal Government*, p. 123.

9 Kenneth O. Morgan, *Bristol and the Atlantic Trade in the Eighteenth Century* (Cambridge: Cambridge University Press, 1993), p. 1; C.M. MacInnes, *Bristol: A Gateway of Empire* (Bristol: Arrowsmith, 1939).

10 See David Hussey, *Coastal and River Trade in Pre-Industrial England: Bristol and Its Region, 1680–1730*, Exeter Maritime Studies (Exeter: Exeter University Press, 2000); David Hussey, 'Metropolis of the West: Bristol and Its Domestic Hinterland, 1680–1731' in Wardley (ed.), *Bristol Histori-cal Resource*. See also David Harris Sacks, *The Widening Gate: Bristol and the Atlantic Economy, 1450–1700* (Berkeley and Oxford: University of California Press, 1991).

11 Philip Ollerenshaw and Peter Wardley, 'Economic Growth and the Busi-ness Community in Bristol since 1840' in Dresser and Ollerenshaw (eds), *Making of Modern Bristol*, pp. 124–5; Brian Atkinson, *Trade Unions in Bristol* (Bristol: Bristol Branch of the Historical Association, 1982), p. 1.

12 Charles Harvey and Jon Press, 'Industrial Change and the Economic Life of Bristol since 1800' in Charles Harvey and Jon Press (eds), *Studies in the Business History of Bristol* (Bristol: Bristol Academic Press, 1988), pp. 2–3 and 8; Peter Malpass and Andy King, *Bristol's Floating Harbour: The First 200 Years* (Bristol: Redcliffe Press, 2009).

13 Charles Harvey and Jon Press, 'Preface' in Harvey and Press (eds), *Busi-ness History*, p. xiv.

14 Ian Archer, Jordan Spencer, Ketih Ramsay, Peter Wardley and Matthew Woollard, 'Unemployment Statistics 1910–1997' in Wardley (ed.), *Bristol Historical Resource*, ch. 4.

15 Meller, *Leisure*.

16 Charles Madge, 'The Propensity to Save in Blackburn and Bristol', *Eco-nomic Journal*, 50:200 (1940), 411.

17 John Stevenson, *British Society 1914–1945* (Harmondsworth: Penguin, 1984), p. 119.

18 Herbert Tout, *The Standard of Living in Bristol* (Bristol: University of Bristol: Arroswmith, 1938), pp. 11 and 24–6.

19 *Report of the Committee Appointed to Inquire into the Condition of the Bristol Poor* (Bristol: P.S. King, 1884), p. 24.

20 *Ibid.*, pp. 26–8.

21 Bristol Medical Officer of Health [hereafter MOH], *Report for 1897*, p. 27.

22 *Condition of the Poor*, pp. 24–5.

23 The National Archives [hereafter TNA], MH 66/1068, 'County Borough of Bristol' Allan C Parsons (Ministry of Health, 1932), p. 27.

24 John Hazlehurst, 'Health Inequalities in Bristol 1918–1939' in Wardley (ed.), *Bristol Historical Resource*, ch. 2.

25 'Census of England and Wales, 1931: County of Gloucester' (London: HMSO, 1933), pp. 16–17.

26 'Census of England and Wales, 1921: County of Gloucester' (London: HMSO, 1923), p. 2; '1931 Census', p. 2; 'Census 1951, England and Wales County Report: Gloucestershire' (London: HMSO, 1954), p. 3.

27 Gorsky, *Patterns of Philanthropy*, p. 21.

28 Frank Borwick (ed.), *Clifton College Annals and Register 1862–1912* (Bristol: Arrowsmith, 1912), pp. 129–30.

29 'Lesser Columbus' (pseudonym) in *Greater Bristol* (London: Pelham, 1893), p. 32.

30 DiGaetano, 'Urban Governance', p. 266.

31 See Jo Manton, *Mary Carpenter and the Children of the Streets* (London: Heinemann Educational, 1976), p. 42.

32 S.T. Coleridge, *An Answer to a Letter to Edward Fox* (Bristol, 1795) cited in Steve Poole, 'To Be a Bristolian: Civic Identity and the Social Order, 1750–1850' in Dresser and Ollerenshaw (eds), *Making of Modern Bristol*, p. 82.

33 *The Annual Register, Or, A View of the History, Politics, and Literature for the Year 1831* (London: J. Dodsley, 1832), pp. 291–5; Geoffrey Amey, *City Under Fire: The Bristol Riots and Aftermath* (London: Lutterworth Press, 1979); James Fawckner Nicholls and John Taylor, *Bristol Past and Present: Civil and Modern History* (Bristol: J.W. Arrowsmith, 1882), pp. 323–8; Poole, 'To Be a Bristolian', p. 85.

34 Madge Dresser and Peter Fleming, *Bristol: Ethnic Minorities and the City 1000–2001* (Chichester: Phillimore, 2007), pp. 146–9.

35 A lack of local chartist activity has been noted in Kieran Kelly and Mike Richardson, 'The Shaping of the Bristol Labour Movement, 1885–1985' in Dresser and Ollerenshaw (eds), *Making of Modern Bristol*, p. 211; John Cannon, *The Chartists in Bristol* (Bristol: Bristol Branch of the Historical Association, 1964), p. 4; Poole, 'To Be a Bristolian', p. 86.

36 Kelly and Richardson, 'Bristol Labour Movement', p. 211.
37 David Large and Robert Whitfield, *The Bristol Trades Council, 1873–1973* (Bristol: Bristol Branch of the Historical Association, 1973), pp. 3–4.
38 Atkinson, *Trade Unions*, pp. 5–7.
39 Kelly and Richardson, 'Bristol Labour Movement', p. 219.
40 See George Campbell Gosling, 'The Patient Contract in Bristol's Voluntary Hospitals, c.1918–1929', *University of Sussex Journal of Contemporary History*, 11 (2007), 10–11.
41 Large and Whitfield, *Bristol Trades Council*, p. 22.
42 *Ibid.*, pp. 22–3.
43 Kelly and Richardson, 'Bristol Labour Movement', p. 220.
44 Archer *et al.*, 'Unemployment Statistics', ch. 4.
45 Kelly and Richardson, 'Bristol Labour Movement', pp. 221–2.
46 Samson Bryher, *An Account of the Labour and Socialist Movement in Bristol* (Bristol: Bristol Labour Weekly, 1929), vol. 1, pp. 24 and 26; vol. 2, pp. 5, 11, 21, 22, 25 and 69, cited in Stephen Yeo, 'A New Life: The Religion of Socialism in Britain, 1883–1896', *History Workshop Journal*, 4:1 (1977), 29–37.
47 Duncan Tanner, *Political Change and the Labour Party, 1900–1918*, 2002 edition (Cambridge: Cambridge University Press, 1990), pp. 298–9; Kelly and Richardson, 'Bristol Labour Movement', p. 212.
48 Large and Whitfield, *Bristol Trades Council*, pp. 17–9 and 23–4.
49 Kelly and Richardson, 'Bristol Labour Movement', p. 222.
50 Ian Archer *et al.*, 'Political Representation and Bristol's Elections 1700–2000' in Wardley (ed.), *Bristol Historical Resource*, ch. 2; Poole, 'To Be a Bristolian', pp. 85–6.
51 Archer *et al.*, 'Political Representations'; 'City Council Chamber Remains Hung', *BBC News*, 6 May 2005, http://news.bbc.co.uk/1/hi/uk_politics/vote_2005/england/4521511.stm, accessed 25 April 2016.
52 Kelly and Richardson, 'Bristol Labour Movement', pp. 222–3.
53 Archer *et al.*, 'Political Representations', ch. 2.
54 Citizen Party, 'Bristol Election Special', October 1947, Bristol Reference Library.
55 Tanner, *Political Change*, p. 299.
56 *Ibid.*, p. 287.
57 Archer *et al.*, 'Political Representations', ch. 2.
58 Martin, 'Managing the Poor', pp. 157–8.
59 *Ibid.*, pp. 157–9; Ian Archer, Jordan Spencer, Ketih Ramsay, Peter Wardley and Matthew Woollard, , 'Poor Law Statistics 1835–1948' in Wardley (ed.), *Bristol Historical Resource*, ch. 3.
60 Martin, 'Managing the Poor', p. 159.

61 *Ibid.*, p. 160.
62 *Ibid.*, pp. 162–78.
63 Parsons, 'Bristol', pp. 6–7.
64 Stanley Hutton, *Bristol and Its Famous Associations* (Bristol: Arrowsmith, 1907), p. 388.
65 *Ibid.*, pp. 396–400; Rohit Barot, *Bristol and the Indian Independence Movement* (Bristol: Bristol Branch of the Historical Association, 1988), pp. 1–7.
66 June Hannam, ' "An Enlarged Sphere of Usefulness": The Bristol Women's Movement, c.1860–1914' in Dresser and Ollerenshaw (eds), *Making of Modern Bristol*, pp. 184–209; Hutton, *Bristol and Its Famous Associations*, pp. 394–6.
67 Meller, *Leisure.*
68 Borwick, *Clifton College Annals*, pp. 134–7.
69 Gorsky, *Patterns of Philanthropy*, p. 231.
70 *Ibid.*
71 Mary Fissell, *Patients, Power, and the Poor in Eighteenth-Century Bristol* (Cambridge: Cambridge University Press, 1991), pp. 74 and 93.
72 Meller, *Leisure.*
73 Roderick Walters, *The Establishment of the Bristol Police Force* (Bristol: Bristol Branch of the Historical Association, 1975), pp. 1 and 6–7; DiGaetano, 'Urban Governance', pp. 266 and 272.
74 Gorsky, *Patterns of Philanthropy*, pp. 222–5; Large, *Municipal Government*, p. 123.
75 DiGaetano, 'Urban Governance', pp. 281–2.
76 David Large and Frances Round, *Public Health in Mid-Victorian Bristol* (Bristol Branch of the Historical Association, 1974); Large, *Municipal Government*, pp. 103–7.
77 Cyril Gibson, *The Bristol School Board 1871–1903* (Bristol Branch of the Historical Association, 1997), pp. 1 and 12; Borwick, *Clifton College Annals*, p. 124.
78 Peter Lamb, *Electricity in Bristol* (Bristol: Bristol Branch of the Historical Association, 1981), p. 3.
79 Hartman Wolfgang Just, *Facts for Bristol: An Exhaustive Collection of Statistical and Other Facts Relating to the City; with Suggestions for Reform on Socialist Principles,* Fabian Tracts, no. 18 (Fabian Society, May 1891), p. 2. For a similar critique see 'Lesser Columbus', *Greater Bristol.*
80 Martin, 'Managing the Poor', p. 165; Madge Dresser, 'People's Housing in Bristol, 1870–1939' in Ian Bild (ed.), *Bristol's Other History* (Bristol: Bristol Broadsides, 1983), pp. 129–60.
81 Clare Hickman, *Therapeutic Landscapes: A History of English Hospital Gardens Since 1800* (Manchester: Manchester University Press, 2013).

82 Nabb, *Bristol Gas Industry*, pp. 1–6.
83 Large, *Municipal Government*, pp. 109–14.
84 Harrison, 'Travel', p. 45.
85 Anne Digby and Nick Bosanquet, 'Doctors and Patients in an Era of National Health Insurance and Private Practice, 1913–1938', *Economic History Review*, 41:1 (1988), 79.
86 *Wright's Bristol Directory* (London: J Wright and Co., 1919), pp. 866–9; *Kelly's (Wright's) Bristol Directory* (London: Kelly's Directories, 1923), pp. 949–52; *Kelly's Directory of Bristol* (London: Kelly's Directories, 1930), pp. 1030–4; *Kelly's Directory of Bristol* (London: Kelly's Directories, 1939), pp. 132–5.
87 Parsons, 'Bristol', p. 11.
88 Bristol MOH, *Report for 1943*; BRO, Bristol Health Committee [hereafter BHC], Minute Book, 1916–1917.
89 BRO, M/BCC/HEA/1/11, BHC Minute Book, Edmund Taylor, 'Maternity and Child Welfare: Note by the Town Clerk' (1917), p. 38.
90 Bristol MOH, *Report*, (1943).
91 D.S. Davies, *The Health of Bristol (City and Port)* (Bristol, 1927), p. 66.
92 Bristol MOH, *Report for 1936*; TNA, MH 79/348, 'Diet and Nutrition: Milk. Investigation into Working Arrangements for Supply to Mothers and Infants under M.C.W. Act' by Dorothy Taylor (Ministry of Health, 1936).
93 Alysa Levene *et al.*, *From Cradle to Grave: Municipal Provision in Interwar England and Wales* (Bern: Peter Lang, 2011), p. 65.
94 Parsons, 'Bristol', 155; Martin Gorsky, ' "For the Treatment of Sick Persons of All Classes": The Transformation of Bristol's Hospital Services, 1918–1939' in Wardley (ed.), *Bristol Historical Resource*, ch. 4.2.
95 Archer *et al.*, 'Unemployment Statistics', ch. 4.
96 Bristol Charity Organization Society, *Report for 1907*, pp. 4–6.
97 *Ibid.*; Bristol Charity Organization Society, *Report for 1908*, p. 20; Bristol Civic League, *Report for 1914*, p. 32; Bristol Civic League for Social Services, *Report for 1927*, p. 14.
98 Bristol Civic League for Social Services, *Report for 1940*, p. 20.
99 Bristol Civic League for Social Services, *Report for 1929*, p. 9.
100 Bristol Civic League for Social Services, *Report for 1937*, p. 8; Bristol Civic League for Social Services, *Report for 1938*, p. 9; Bristol Civic League for Social Services, *Report for 1940*, p. 2.
101 Bristol Civic League for Social Services, *Report for 1937*, p. 9.
102 Bristol Civic League for Social Services, *Report for 1941*, pp. 6–7; Bristol Civic League for Social Services, *Report for 1942*, pp. 4–6.
103 DiGaetano, 'Urban Governance'.

104 Gorsky, *Patterns of Philanthropy*, p. 234.
105 For something closer to a comprehensive survey of the city's hospitals in the period, see George Campbell Gosling, 'Charity and Change in the Mixed Economy of Healthcare in Bristol, 1918–1948', unpublished PhD thesis, Oxford Brookes University, 2011, pp. 61–93.
106 Gorsky, 'Bristol's Hospital Services', ch. 5.1.
107 BRI, *Reports for 1921–1938*; BGH, *Reports for 1921–1938*; Bristol Homeopathic Hospital, *Report for 1937*, p. 26.
108 G. Munro Smith, *A History of the Bristol Royal Infirmary* (Bristol: Arrowsmith, 1917), pp. 5–9.
109 Charles Clarke, *Bristol Royal Infirmary: A Personal Study Written to Commemorate the First 250 Years, 1735–1985* (Bristol: Portishead Press, 1985), p. 3; C. Bruce Perry, *Voluntary Medical Institutions* (Bristol: Bristol Branch of the Historical Association, 1984), p. 2; Charles Saunders, *The United Bristol Hospitals* (Bristol: United Bristol Hospitals, 1965), p. 12.
110 F.K. Prochaska, *Philanthropy and the Hospitals of London: The King's Fund, 1897–1990* (Oxford: Clarendon Press, 1992), p. 2; Gorsky, 'Bristol's Hospital Services'; Mary Fissell, 'Charity Universal? Institutions and Moral Reform in Eighteenth-Century Bristol' in Lee Davison, Tim Hitchcock, Tim Keirn and Robert Shoemaker (eds), *Still The Grumbling Hive: The Response to Social and Economic Problems in England, 1689–1750* (Stroud: St Martin's Press, 1992), p. 126.
111 Clarke, *Bristol Royal Infirmary*, p. 27; Gorsky, 'Bristol's Hospital Services'.
112 University of Bristol Special Collections [hereafter BSC], DM980 (30), 'Bristol Hospitals Commission, Bristol Hospitals Fund Evidence, Appendix 1' (1941), pp. 1–2.
113 BRI, *Reports*. For more on the finances of the Infirmary, see Gorsky, 'Bristol's Hospital Services', ch. 3.
114 Saunders, *United Bristol Hospitals*, p. 16.
115 Bryan Little, *The City and County of Bristol: A Study in Atlantic Civilisation* (London: SR Publishers, 1954), p. 277.
116 BGH, *Reports*; BRI, *Reports*.
117 John Odery Symes, *A Short History of the Bristol General Hospital* (Bristol: J. Wright and Co., 1932), p. 1.
118 *Ibid.*, 10; Archer *et al.*, 'Political Representations'.
119 Bruce Perry, *Voluntary Medical Institutions*, p. 6.
120 V. Zachary Cope *et al.*, 'Hospital Survey: The Hospital Services of the South-Western Area' (London: HMSO, 1945), p. 178.
121 Saunders, *United Bristol Hospitals*, pp. 18–19.
122 Cope *et al.*, 'Hospital Survey', p. 178.
123 'BRI Report' (1921), p. 11.

124 Lindsay Granshaw, ' "Fame and Fortune by Means of Bricks and Mortar":
    The Medical Profession and Specialist Hospitals in Britain, 1800–1948' in
    Lindsay Granshaw and Roy Porter (eds), *The Hospital in History* (London:
    Routledge, 1989), pp. 199–220.
125 Charles Saunders, *The Bristol Eye Hospital* (Bristol: United Bristol Hospi-
    tals, 1960), p. 10; V.J. Marmion, *The Bristol Eye Hospital: A Monograph*
    (Bristol, 1987), p. 6.
126 Cope *et al.*, 'Hospital Survey', p. 179.
127 Bristol Orthopaedic Hospital, *Reports for 1921–1930*.
128 Bristol Orthopaedic Hospital, *Report for 1930*, p. 2.
129 John Lyes, *Bristol 1927–1933* (Bristol: Bristol Branch of the Historical
    Association, 2004), p. 15; Bruce Perry, *Voluntary Medical Institutions*, p.
    19; Bristol MOH, *Report for 1930*, p. 42.
130 Bruce Perry, *Voluntary Medical Institutions*, pp. 15–6; Charles Saunders,
    The Bristol Royal Hospital for Sick Children (Bristol: United Bristol Hospi-
    tals, 1961), p. 9.
131 Bristol Children's Hospital, *Report for 1920*, p. 3.
132 Cope *et al.*, 'Hospital Survey', p. 178.
133 *Ibid.*, p. 26.
134 Wellcome Library, Archives and Manuscripts, SA/MWF/C.22:Box 20,
    Medical Women's Federation, Section II: Hospitals founded by women,
    Bristol: Walker Dunbar.
135 Saunders, *United Bristol Hospitals*, p. 79.
136 Cope *et al.*, 'Hospital Survey', p. 26.
137 *Ibid.*, pp. 178–9.
138 For more on this institution and others, see George Campbell Gosling,
    'The Birth of the Pregnant Patient-Consumer? Payment, Paternalism and
    Maternity Hospitals in Early Twentieth-Century England' in Jennifer
    Evans and Ciara Meehan, *Perceptions of Pregnancy from the Seventeenth to
    Twentieth Century* (London: Palgrave Macmillan, 2016).
139 Reprinted in the *Western Daily Press*, cited in Charles Saunders, *The Bristol
    Maternity Hospital* (Bristol: United Bristol Hospitals, 1961), p. 9.
140 *Ibid.*, pp. 12–3; Cope *et al.*, 'Hospital Survey', p. 32; Bristol MOH, *Report
    for 1930*, p. 42; Lyes, *Bristol 1927–1933*, p. 8.
141 BCM, 13 September 1921, 'Report of the Health Committee, 30 August
    1921'.
142 BCM, 10 October 1933, 'Report of the Health Committee, 26 September
    1933'; Saunders, *Maternity Hospital*, p. 18; Lyes, *Bristol 1927–1933*, p. 17;
    Bruce Perry, *Voluntary Medical Institutions*, p. 17.
143 Saunders, *Maternity Hospital*, p. 17.
144 Bristol Children's Hospital, *Reports*.

145 John Lyes, *Bristol 1920–1926* (Bristol: Bristol Branch of the Historical Association, 2003), pp. 14 and 29.

146 Bruce Perry, *Voluntary Medical Institutions*, p. 14; Saunders, *United Bristol Hospitals*, p. 58; Bristol Homeopathic Hospital, *Report for 1937*, pp. 7–8; Cope *et al.*, 'Hospital Survey', p. 26.

147 BRO, 41171/Mgt/Co/4, Cossham Memorial Hospital, 'Charity Commissioner correspondence, 1928–1938, Settlement of the Estate of Handel Cossham deceased, 1891'.

148 'Famous Bristol Landmarks 8: Cossham Hospital Tower', *Bristol Evening Post*, 19 June 1954.

149 Cossham Memorial Hospital, *Report for 1935*, p. 5.

150 Cossham Memorial Hospital, *Report for 1931*, p. 6; Cossham Memorial Hospital, *Report for 1935*, p. 6.

151 Cossham Memorial Hospital, *Report for 1931*, p. 6; Cossham Memorial Hospital, *Report for 1936*, p. 5.

152 Ruth Hodgkinson, *The Origins of the National Health Service: The Medical Services of the New Poor Law, 1834–1871* (London: Wellcome Historical Medical Library, 1967).

153 Parsons, 'Bristol, p. 149.

154 Cope *et al.*, 'Hospital Survey', p. 34; S. Datta, 'Report of the Medical Officer, Stapleton Institution' in *Bristol MOH Report for 1937*, pp. 164–5.

155 J.A. Lanson, 'Report of the Medical Officer, Eastville Institution' in *Bristol MOH Report for 1937*, p. 166.

156 BRO, M/BCC/SOW/4/2, 'Social Welfare Committee – Stapleton and Eastville Minutes', 1 July 1938; Bristol MOH, *Report for 1930*, p. 145.

157 Bristol MOH, *Report for 1943*, p. 36.

158 Parsons, 'Bristol', p. 135; Bristol MOH, *Report for 1930*, p. 42; Gorsky, 'Bristol's Hospital Services'; Cope *et al.*, 'Hospital Survey', p. 25.

159 Parsons, 'Bristol', p. 129; BCM, 8 April 1930, BHC, *Report*, 1 April 1930.

160 BHC Minutes, 1 January 1930.

161 H.J. Maggs, 'Report of the Chairman of the Health Committee', 31 May 1932 in BHC Minutes, 14 June 1932.

162 Barbara Buchanan, '2,600 Babies Start Their Lives Here Every Year', *Bristol Evening World*, 19 January 1943.

163 Bristol MOH, *Report for 1927*, p. 71; BCM, 9 April 1924 'Report of the Health Committee', 1 April 1924; Bristol MOH, *Report for 1924*, p. 13.

164 Bristol MOH, *Report for 1920*, p. 58.

165 'New Corporation Hospital at Bristol', *British Medical Journal*, 29 July 1899.

166 Bristol MOH, *Report for 1927*, p. 72; Cope *et al.*, 'Hospital Survey', p. 33; Gorsky, 'Bristol's Hospital Services', ch. 4.2; Maggs, 'Report of the Chairman of the Health Committee'.
167 Bristol MOH, *Report for 1924*, pp. 12–16; B.A.I. Peters, 'Report of the Medical Superintendent, Ham Green Hospital and Sanatorium' in Bristol MOH, *Report for 1937*, pp. 140–1; Bristol MOH, *Report for 1924*, p. 59.
168 Bristol MOH, *Report for 1933*, p. 113.
169 Bristol MOH, *Report for 1930*, pp. 42–3; James Briggs, *The History of Frenchay Hospital* (Bristol: Monica Britton Hall of Medical History, 1994), p. 15.
170 Bristol MOH, *Report for 1942*, p. 74; Cope *et al.*, 'Hospital Survey', p. 33.
171 Levene *et al.*, *Cradle to Grave*, p. 65.

3

Payment and the sick poor

In 1935 Sir Alan Garrett Anderson, son of the pioneer of women in medicine, Elizabeth Garrett Anderson, was elected Conservative MP for the City of London. A year later he spoke in a parliamentary debate on the nation's voluntary hospitals:

> We have been told that they are passing through a lean time and are in competition with the municipal hospitals, but I demur to both those statements. The hospitals are always short of cash, because they are doing a great and expanding work, but they are getting enormous voluntary support from the whole class who will be treated in the hospitals all over the country. I do not think that 'a lean time' is the correct expression. They are being more and more useful as the community learns the importance of health, and the provision of health is getting more and more expensive. During the last 10 or 15 years there have come into being more and more departments which are like telescopes to look inside us and prevent disease before it begins. Those departments are very expensive, and that is why the balance sheet is difficult to balance; and, without help from all the patients, the hospitals would, of course, have broken down, and there would have been a great disturbance of the whole health service.[1]

Put plainly, the interwar era was a time when hospitals could do more but afford less. In this context, we can see a reluctant adoption of patient payments as the chosen means to survive. The question this prompts is the extent to which philanthropy as the organising principle of the voluntary hospital system was undermined or even abandoned by this decision.

Charity was not crowded out by the expanding public sector in the early twentieth century, but neither did it continue unchanged. As discussed in the previous chapter, the voluntary sector expanded in partnership with the state. In Bristol as elsewhere, the voluntary hospitals were just one area in which this was the case. However, the relationship between the voluntary hospitals and the state was not always an easy one. The hospitals' involvement in meeting the demands of the First World War was the most bruising example of government being ready to ask more but unwilling to pick up the tab. The financial strains were exaggerated by a challenging postwar economic climate, increasing demand and ever greater technological requirements in hospital medicine. As the new decade of the 1920s beckoned there were genuine grounds for optimism in the growing capabilities of hospital medicine, yet placing the work of the voluntary hospitals on a sound financial footing was an even harder task than usual. A new settlement was required – a new contract with the traditional working-class patient, represented by the character of 'George' in the 1948 cartoon *Your Very Good Health* – in which payment was to become an important feature.

The fundamental question this chapter seeks to answer is whether the incorporation of payment into this revised patient contract amounted to an abandonment of philanthropy. The appointment of hospital almoners to conduct what was effectively a means-test served as a double-safeguard. First, it allowed the hospital to grant reductions and exemptions to those unable to pay, ensuring this did not become a barrier to access. Second, along with the setting of income limits, the assessment of the almoner was a mechanism for weeding out those of the middle and upper classes who were not considered appropriate cases for medical charity. Beyond mere safeguards, however, the new mechanisms and rituals of payment came to reinforce philanthropy in a variety of ways.

Systems of admission

Prior to the First World War, Bristol's voluntary hospitals were typical in operating two well-established systems for admission: subscriber's tickets and 'receiving day'. In Mary Fissell's study of the eighteenth-century origins of the Bristol (later Royal) Infirmary, she discussed the former, emphasising its characteristics of dominant philanthropist and passive recipient. According to this arrangement, the Bristol Infirmary was founded and primarily maintained by charitable donations, in return for which subscribers were entitled to nominate deserving sick individuals for admission. This 'new channel for paternalism' was purchased at the rate of two guineas a year for one inpatient and up to three outpatients at a time.[2] Although as many as a third of subscribers never made use of this entitlement in the Bristol Infirmary's first century, it was important both for patients, because a subscriber's ticket was necessary for all but emergency admissions, and for maintaining 'networks of patronage'.[3]

As Fissell has explained, 'the recommendation from a hospital supporter required by a prospective patient' was 'a form of social exchange in a face-to-face society. The hospital provided an arena for the mediation of social power, both directly through individual patronage, and symbolically through civic ritual and display'.[4] This face-to-face encounter would often be with someone familiar to the individual through 'residential proximity, employment' or 'religious affiliation'.[5] It was an 'articulation of social difference' between these self-styled 'stewards of the poor' and the recipients who had to prove themselves deserving not only of medical treatment but also capable of 'moral reform'.[6] The subscriber was therefore a powerful figure in this 'gift relationship', discriminating between those suitable for hospital treatment and 'the less worthy paupers who resorted to the workhouse'.[7] A fictional portrait of the system appeared in Elizabeth Gaskell's 1848 novel *Mary Barton*, with its subtitle 'A Tale of Manchester Life':

'If you please, sir,' said a servant, entering the room, 'here's one of the mill people wanting to see you; his name is Wilson, he says.'

'I'll come to him directly; stay, tell him to come here.'

Amy danced off into the conservatory which opened out of the room, before the gaunt, pale, unwashed, unshaven weaver was ushered in. There he stood at the door sleeking his hair with old country habit, and every now and then stealing a glance round at the splendour of the apartment.

'Well, Wilson, and what you want to-day, man?'

'Please, sir, Davenport's ill of the fever, and I'm come to know if you've got an Infirmary order for him?'

'Davenport – Davenport; who is the fellow? I don't know the name.'

'He's worked in your factory better nor three years, sir.'

'Very likely; I don't pretend to know the names of the men I employ; that I leave to the overlooker. So he's ill, eh?'

'Ay, sir, he's very bad; we want to get him in at the Fever Wards.'

'I doubt if I've an in-patient's order to spare at present; but I'll give you an out-patient's and welcome.'

So saying, he rose up, unlocked a drawer, pondered a minute, and then gave Wilson an out-patient's order.

Meanwhile, the younger Mr Carson had ended his review, and began to listen to what was going on. He finished his breakfast, got up, and pulled five shillings out of his pocket, which he gave to Wilson as he passed him, for the 'poor fellow.'[8]

By the early twentieth century, there was significant criticism of the recipient's powerlessness in this relationship: 'Can you imagine the feelings of the dissenting agricultural labourer in a small village who has to go to the vicar for a subscriber's letter? Or those of the village socialist who has to submit to a political lecture from the squire before he can get one?'[9]

This system was not particular to the Bristol Infirmary and became the standard means of accessing services as the voluntary hospital system expanded through the eighteenth and nineteenth centuries.[10] In the latter, however, admission directly by doctors increasingly became an alternative, including at the Bristol Infirmary. This system, where patients would come to the hospital on a 'receiving day' and be seen by a doctor, was the only means of being admitted to the Bristol Royal Hospital for Sick Children and Women from its foundation in 1866.[11] 'Enough that a child be sick and poor', the institution's annual reports declared, 'it will be admitted provided there be an empty bed and that the Medical Officers consider the case a suitable one for admission to the hospital'.[12] By doing so, they were adhering to the principle Dr William Marsden established in 1828 in founding the Royal Free Hospital in London, that 'destitution and disease should alone be the passport for obtaining free and instant relief'.[13] In this alternative, however, even with medical examination replacing the moral subjectivity of the recommendation, the patient remained in an essentially passive role.

For most voluntary hospitals in Bristol, however, admission by means of the subscriber recommendation system continued into the twentieth century. Whereas the subscriber ticket was being phased out of many voluntary hospitals around the turn of the century, those hospitals in Bristol, alongside others including the Birmingham Infirmary and Guy's Hospital, 'retained it in the belief that the issue of subscribers' letters was necessary to sustain the enthusiasm of charitable supporters'. This was an important consideration at a time of declining subscriber income, as noted by Gorsky, Mohan and Powell for the voluntary hospitals, and by Daunton for associational voluntarism more widely.[14] Recommendations also continued at the Radcliffe Infirmary in Oxford, where subscribers' notes known as 'Turns' made one guinea exchangeable for the admission of one inpatient or four outpatients until 1926.[15] In some rare cases, such as the Saturday Fund in Nottingham, it was not until 1938 that subscriber recommendations were abandoned.[16]

Over the 1920s most hospitals gradually replaced recommendations with a new arrangement, whereby admission became an entirely medical matter but payment was increasingly a term of that admission. Payment by patients was not entirely unknown before the twentieth century, as Jonathan Reinarz has demonstrated with a number of examples from eighteenth- and nineteenth-century Birmingham.[17] However, it was not until the start of the 1920s that it became the norm and ingrained in both hospital administration and patient experience. In place of a subscriber judging deservingness, a medical social worker, known in our period as the Lady Almoner, carried out an assessment. It was her task to determine both what further support was necessary and what would be an appropriate financial contribution to ask. The two ways to avoid paying the almoner were either to be deemed unable to pay, something beyond the control of the individual patient, or to be a member of a hospital contributory scheme. This would involve paying a weekly subscription of perhaps two or three pence from weekly wages into a workplace or local fund, the scheme would then cover a contribution on behalf of the patient if admitted.

The recent literature on the pre-NHS hospital sector has rightly given a prominent place to such schemes.[18] They have been characterised as becoming 'an essential element of the British hospital system' in the interwar decades, enabling 'renewed hospital expansion.'[19] Certainly, they were a notable change and provided a useful new income stream – but they are not themselves the whole story. As Martin Gorsky and John Mohan calculate, by the mid-1930s hospital contributory schemes accounted for something in the region of one-third of income for large hospitals across Britain, more than double the amount coming from direct patient payments.[20] This does not mean, however, that twice as many patients were contributory scheme members as not. Exemptions or reductions regularly granted to non-members, as well as grants made to the hospitals by contributory schemes separately from the payments on behalf of their members when hospitalised, mean there is no direct correlation to be drawn between the number of patients in each category and the income derived from them.

In Bristol we see contributory schemes only gradually established over three decades. The first schemes were small workplace ones, not accompanied by a city-wide scheme until 1927 when the Bristol Medical Institutions Contributory Scheme (BMICS) was established. It was hoped this would bring the level of membership in Bristol up to that of the movement's leading lights; yet a decade later campaigners could still point enviously to cities like Sheffield and Liverpool where membership was roughly between one-third and a half of the whole population (including the dependants expected to be covered by the head of the household), and Birmingham where it was well over half. A rival central scheme, the Bristol Hospitals Fund (BHF), was set up in 1939 under the closer control of the hospitals themselves, which does appear to have closed the gap. In the early 1940s, combined membership of the BHF and the Bristol Hospital Contributors League, which brought together the BMICS and the independent workplace schemes, was in the region of 150,000 – more than one-third of the city's population at the time. This proportion was significantly greater than in nearby Cardiff although far less than in Swansea, which was home to the biggest hospital contributory scheme in Wales. There were, therefore, two decades during which it was the norm for patients to pay something to the hospital before Bristol's population adopted a mass-scale membership of the contributory schemes in the 1940s. While the contributory schemes should not be dismissed, they should also not be treated as synonymous with the patient experience in those final decades before the introduction of the NHS. Of greater importance were the more quickly established direct patient payment schemes.

The rest of this chapter will examine the workings of and relationship between these two parallel systems for working-class patients and potential patients making a contribution. Above all, the two will be shown as alternative arrangements for the same act: not buying medical care or even gaining admission, but rather for working-class patients themselves to be enlisted as charitable donors to the hospital.

Patient payment schemes in Bristol

Payment in the voluntary hospitals

In the summer of 1921, in response to the financial difficulties of the years immediately following the First World War, the city's first direct payment scheme was jointly introduced at the Bristol Royal Infirmary and the Bristol General Hospital, side-lining the nominally continued subscriber's tickets. Under this system admission was essentially a clinical decision, but the patient was then expected to contribute towards the cost of their maintenance. These new arrangements were reported in the *Bristol Times and Mirror*:

(1) In-patients, with the exception of necessitous cases, will be charged 21s. per week towards the cost of their maintenance.

(2) Out-patients, with the exception of necessitous cases, will be charged a registration fee of 6d. for each attendance, and an additional 6d. for medicine or dressings, etc., when supplied. X-ray, electrical and massage treatment to be charged for specially, according to the cost.

(3) Insured patients will be required to bring a note from their panel doctor stating that hospital out-patient treatment is necessary, and they will be charged the same rate as other patients.[21]

By December of that year these arrangements had been replicated at the Bristol Eye Hospital, and it was later to become the model for the Bristol Homeopathic Hospital.[22] The patient payment scheme introduced at the Bristol Royal Hospital for Sick Children and Women differed in both its rate of contribution and its geographical qualification. Bristol's Children's Hospital had never taken notes of recommendation, sharing the belief at the Birmingham Women's Hospital that women should not need 'to explain their complaints to anyone but a medical gentleman'.[23] In accordance with this ethos it had previously admitted children up to the age of thirteen free and women 'according to their means'.[24] Under the new arrangements, however, a weekly contribution of five shillings was asked of patients living within a twenty-five mile radius of Bristol, and this was doubled for non-local patients, with the burden of patients from South Wales cited as a factor.[25]

The standard rate of one guinea per week had been introduced at the Norfolk and Norwich Hospital only a year before the joint scheme in

Bristol, and this was taken as the template.[26] One guinea was generally said by the hospitals to be significantly less than the average cost of providing treatment; which the Homeopathic Hospital claimed in 1937 to be £3 3s 4d per week.[27] Yet a guinea was also a significant amount to pay, twice what the average working-class family in the late 1930s spent on a week's rent and two-thirds of that on food.[28] In Bristol in the 1920s it would have been around a third the weekly wage of a shipbuilding labourer and half that of a building or engineering labourer.[29] The local press echoed a joint sub-committee of the two institutions in presenting exemptions from the standard rate of contribution as being for 'really necessitous cases' only.[30] This perhaps contributed to the long-standing perception that 'the contribution was a form of compulsory payment'.[31] However, in practice, exemptions from and reductions to patient payments were extensive.

The exemptions and reductions offered by the almoner allowed the Bristol Royal Infirmary to claim that 'no patient who is financially unable to make a contribution' was expected or even 'asked to do so'.[32] The level of full or partial exemption from contribution was vast. If universally upheld, the new payment scheme would have generated over £10,000 in its first year; the actual figure was £2,968.[33] Although this more than doubled the following year, the degree of exemption remained high enough for Labour Alderman Frank Sheppard, the long-serving deputy then chairman of the city's municipal health committee, to tell the institution's governors it 'clearly showed that they had not received payment from those who were not in a position to make it'. He emphasised this point 'because of the misunderstanding which had arisen over the contribution of a guinea a week'.[34] No doubt this confusion had been aided by the hospitals' using the language of *charges* to announce the scheme.[35] Meanwhile, at the Bristol Homeopathic Hospital in 1937, the work of the almoner's department was said to have 'progressed satisfactorily', largely due to an increase in the number of patients who 'were either without means or only able to contribute very little towards the One Guinea per week contribution asked for, in the General Wards'.[36] Treating those who could not afford to pay, rather than generating higher income from those who could, was the marker of success.

Figures 3.1 and 3.2 show the proportion of patients receiving such exemptions and reductions at the Bristol Royal Infirmary and the

Bristol General Hospital respectively. They cover the period from the first full year of the payment scheme until reported figures do not allow for such distinctions. For both, it should be noted that payments on behalf of patients are included as well as those directly by the patients themselves. Therefore contributory schemes, as well as charitable or public bodies sponsoring patients, are an unmeasured and inseparable proportion of that category. From the outset, it was noted at both hospitals that local workplace schemes accounted for the majority of payments of one guinea or more.[37] Meanwhile, those admitted entirely free became a smaller proportion of those admitted to both. However, while Cherry has asserted that patient payments became 'generalized' over this period,[38] in Bristol's two major general voluntary hospitals at least, free and subsidised treatment continued to be a major feature of the institution.

The hospitals therefore admitted a mix of patients throughout the interwar years as the new system bedded in and payment became the norm. Some were passed free. This category continued, although it

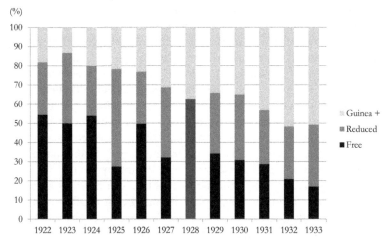

Figure 3.1 Proportions of patients paying different rates at the Bristol Royal Infirmary, 1922–33
Note: Figures given for 1928 do not allow for a distinction between reductions and exemptions.

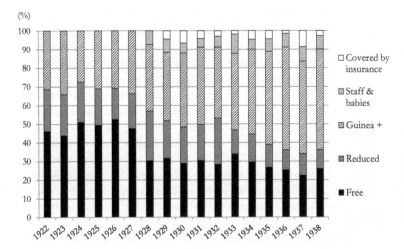

Figure 3.2 Proportions of patients paying different rates at the Bristol General Hospital, 1922–38

halved at the Bristol General Hospital and fell further and quicker at the Bristol Royal Infirmary, where patients were more likely to pay at a reduced rate instead. Those cases where the institution received the full guinea payment or more (either from the patient directly or on their behalf) had only grown to approximately half of all inpatients by the mid-1930s. From this time onwards it grew further, although those receiving admission free or at a reduced rate remained above 40 per cent even after the two hospitals amalgamated in 1939. The variable but consistently significant proportion of patients in these free and reduced payment categories was said to be determined largely by the state of the local economy, increasing at times of high unemployment.[39]

This high rate of free admission cannot be dismissed as a consequence of contributory scheme membership being smaller in Bristol than some other cities, as seen from Nottingham, where scheme members accounted for 60 per cent of patients. The Nottingham General Hospital fell between Bristol's two general voluntary hospitals, with one in five deemed unable to pay and admitted free.[40] Meanwhile the figure was one in ten at the city's Eye Hospital, despite historian Nick Hayes judging the institution 'financially punctilious' and eager to limit free admissions.[41] In the annual reports of Bristol hospitals, almoners repeatedly claimed that 'inability to make a contribution' had never led to a patient being refused treatment, and that offers had been rejected when 'the money was needed in the patient's home, or to tide over the period that might intervene between leaving the Infirmary and a return to work'.[42] This was seen in action retrospectively in 1925 when one patient's payments at five shillings a week were refunded after it was brought to the House Committee's attention 'that it was a very great hardship to her to pay anything'.[43] However, it should be noted that this example could be used to support either the argument that payments were declined or that the assessments may not have guaranteed that all individuals unable to pay were admitted free. Either way, it is clear payment was not a fixed price but was constantly negotiated and renegotiated on the basis of the patient's circumstances.

Across the city's voluntary hospitals, therefore, we see a mixed system developing, according to which contributory scheme members and other funded patients were increasingly admitted to the general wards alongside philanthropically subsidised patients. This description fits those paying the full guinea rate, which was approximately only one-third of the full cost of maintenance, as well as those admitted free or at a reduced rate.

Payment at the municipal hospitals

It is easy to cast interwar municipal hospitals as forerunners of the National Health Service, providing tax-funded medical services to the whole community and making important strides towards a more integrated and co-ordinated hospital system.[44] Not always, however, services free at the point of use. A similar payment system to that of the voluntary hospitals was also to be found at Bristol's municipal Southmead Hospital. An early 1930s Ministry of Health survey noted that 'if treated in the general wards the fee is £2.2.0', twice the full rate at the voluntary hospitals, with higher fees again for middle-class patients in private rooms (discussed in the next chapter).[45] The principle underpinning this gradation of payment was said to be 'that the sick poor would have first claim upon the accommodation at Southmead, but any citizen would have the right to apply for a bed at the Hospital, subject to the condition of paying all or part of the cost, if able'.[46]

Little has been written in previous studies to suggest how widespread this approach was in public infirmaries. However, Doyle has noted 'the charging of non-pauper paying patients £1 10s per week', a significantly lower rate, at a similar institution in Middlesbrough.[47] He has also found paying patients alongside paupers in the poor law infirmaries of Leeds and Sheffield from the mid-1920s, prominent amongst whom were maternity cases and hospital contributory scheme members.[48] What this suggests is that there was likely a now-forgotten practice of pre-NHS municipal hospitals charging patients akin to that of the voluntary sector. Indeed, under the 1929 Local Government Act it was 'the duty of the Corporation ... to recover the cost of treatment from all patients who are able to pay'.[49] However, the public hospitals in Bristol seem to have gone far beyond their legal duty and the higher rates charged suggests they may even have embraced this more eagerly than their voluntary counterparts.

The matter was addressed further by the city's municipal health committee in 1933, in a discussion of Southmead's expanding specialist maternity provision. The Liberal chairman, H.J. Maggs, said the rates charged at Southmead were still low enough to show the development of its services as a municipal general hospital was intended for the treatment of what he called 'the hospital class of patient'.

> It must be stressed again that in the extension of facilities at Southmead the accommodation was for the class of patient who could not afford treatment other than in a hospital; your Committee were not considering any other class. That it is this class who are availing themselves of the facilities at Southmead is shown by an analysis of the maternity cases admitted in 1932. The scale of charges are such that a man (with wife and one child) who earns more than £1 19s 2d per week (net income) is assessed to pay the full cost of treatment. Approximately 56 per cent. of the cases admitted in 1932 fell below this standard and 30 per cent. (approximately) were unable to pay anything at all, and were given free treatment. There were several more on the borderline, and although assessed to pay the full charge they were unable to do so.[50]

Reflecting the similarities between the voluntary and municipal hospital payment schemes, Southmead appointed an almoner in April 1937.[51] The figures in her annual reports to the city's Medical Officer of Health (given in figure 3.3) demonstrate that the mix of patients paying

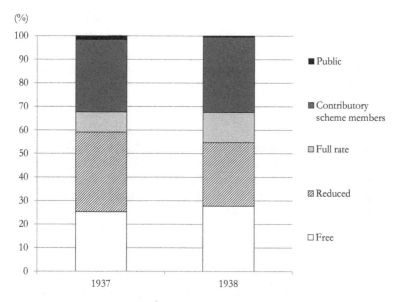

Figure 3.3 Proportions of patients paying different rates at Southmead
Hospital, 1937–38

different rates was strikingly similar to the voluntary hospitals. There
are two differences we can note. One is that payments from contributory schemes and public bodies are given separately from those patients
paying the full rate here. What this different method of recording the
figures reveals supports the assertion of the voluntary hospitals that
the majority of those paying the full rate were contributory scheme
members. We might expect them to be patients in the voluntary hospitals, which had a far better-established working relationship with the
contributory schemes, yet at Southmead they accounted for nearly one-
third of patients. For contributory scheme members in Bristol, as in
London and elsewhere, it would appear the development of maternity
and other services made Southmead an acceptable alternative to either
of its voluntary counterparts, despite the ongoing stigma of having been
a workhouse infirmary.[52]

The other difference is the greater proportion of patients paying at a
reduced rate. However, this is easily explained by the fact that the full

rate was two guineas instead of the one asked for in the voluntary hospitals. As such, it is clear that the interwar years saw a common system of means-tested financial contribution (although not commercial fees) established in general wards across the public/voluntary hospital divide in Bristol.

Reluctant change

Although the reasons for introducing such schemes were varied, there does not appear to have been any great degree of zealotry about taking a step towards a commercial model of provision, even from those at the hospitals most actively pressing for the introduction of payment schemes.[53] At the Bristol Royal Infirmary the Faculty were concerned that 'the admission of the cases for payment would give them priority and would thus still further diminish the accommodation for the suffering poor'.[54] When five honorary staff members addressed the institution's General Committee in 1920, they explained that they were 'merely anxious that the long Waiting Lists of Patients should be admitted, it being evident that, at present, this could only be done if some form of payment was received from those who could afford it'.[55] As such, financial rather than ideological motivations were paramount.[56]

The financial imperative to consider the introduction of pay beds was considerable. A 1919 committee meeting had 'unanimously agreed that at present it was impossible to increase the number of free beds at all' at the Bristol Royal Infirmary, 'and that the provision of paying beds should be considered at once'.[57] A year later the number of beds was restricted to 238, only to be increased if the full cost of the bed could be paid to the hospital.[58] The *Bristol Times and Mirror* reported 'the important new direction' as one the hospital's governors had 'been forced to take', which was 'inevitable if the work were to be continued in any degree according to need'.[59] There were reformers elsewhere who advocated payment on more than strictly financial grounds. Though when Robert Hogarth called for a payment scheme in Nottingham, 'not simply a matter of maximizing income' but to encourage a collective sense of ownership and of entitlement to treatment, he found he was voicing an unpopular opinion.[60] For most of those engaged in establishing hospital payment schemes, the reason for doing so was overwhelmingly one of financial necessity.

The Lady Almoner

When payment schemes were introduced, the task of achieving that difficult balance between generating new income and maintaining a philanthropic ethos typically fell to a new figure in the voluntary hospitals: the Lady Almoner. Yet she is a figure often found in the background if not entirely omitted from the recent historical literature. Former almoners writing on their profession's history include Angela Simmons' postgraduate work, in which she located early pioneers firmly within a late-Victorian social context.[61] Phyllis Willmott's narrative of the first fifty years of the almoner profession (until 1945) emphasised the role of various London-based committees in building the profession.[62] Meanwhile, some historians have also tentatively turned their attention to the almoner.

Keir Waddington located the initial introduction of almoners in London firmly within the late nineteenth-century debate around out-patient abuse.[63] Lynsey Cullen has added to this by conducting the first rigorous investigation of the archival records of an almoner's department, using this source to better understand the patient intake and range of diseases, as well as the contribution of the almoner to their care. Her focus was restricted to the first almoner, Miss Mary Stewart, appointed at the Royal Free Hospital in London in 1895 and retiring in 1899.[64] Rona Dougall and Chris Nottingham's work on Scottish social work within the NHS, identifying it as an 'insecure profession', is unusual for bringing the story so far into the twentieth century.[65] For the most part the limited literature on the almoner profession remains heavily focused on its earliest days and on London. What this misses is the rapid and widespread growth of the profession beyond the capital in the interwar years. One historian to venture into this territory is Elaine Thomson, describing the Edinburgh Hospital for Women and Children's almoner as 'keeping working-class patients under surveillance in their own homes', reflecting her role at a very specific type of voluntary hospital.[66] Another local case study by Barry Doyle has found the Leeds General Infirmary to have appointed an almoner in 1910, rather earlier than most provincial towns, with appointments in other hospitals following in the 1920s. While they balanced financial and social support roles, their counterparts in nearby Sheffield adopted a greater focus on after-care in the later 1930s.[67]

While these contributions are very welcome, they fall far short of providing a coherent picture of the profession as a whole across Britain and over the half-century before the introduction of the NHS changed their function fundamentally. It is therefore worth briefly considering how the profession was understood at the time.

The almoner profession: finance and social work

A common theme running through the contemporary literature on the almoner was a tension between the social work side of the almoner's role and their involvement with patient payment schemes. Dorothy Manchée, almoner at St Mary's Hospital in London, wrote a pseudo-autobiographical novel which she called *Whatever Does an Almoner Do?* She wrote it, in part, in the hope of 'combating the unfortunate and incorrect impression of many lay people that "she interviews patients' relatives about fees"!'[68] In one passage, where the almoner is talking to a young woman considering the profession, the author takes the opportunity to dispel some common misconceptions:

'Being an Almoner,' Ann Clavering explained, 'is rather like being a Universal Aunt. Everyone in the hospital and many outside come with their troubles and problems for us to help solve. We find homes for babies and jobs for cripples; extra food for the hungry and extra money for the needy; glasses for those who can't see and wheel chairs for those who can't walk. Sometimes we are asked for paper carriers and drawing pins! The man-in-the-street usually thinks we collect money for the hospital, and that's about the only job we don't do!'

'I thought you asked people what they earned and told them what to pay for their treatment,' said Yvonne in astonishment.

'The Almoners in some hospitals do so because they believe that they know the patients best and so can be more fair to them, but at this hospital we don't even do that. We're just here to help people get the best advantage from their hospital visits.'[69]

This was one of a number of books published on the eve of the NHS seeking to clarify the role of the hospital almoner and distance her from financial assessment, perhaps prompted by concern that if the profession was too closely associated with patient payments it would be seen as superfluous under the new system.

From the appointment of the first hospital almoner, the focus was on the financial side of the role. When the Charity Organisation Society

(COS) caseworker Mary Stewart was appointed, she was given three duties: to prevent the 'abuse' of admission being given to 'persons able to pay for medical treatment'; to refer the 'destitute' to the Poor Law; and to encourage those between the two to join 'Provident Dispensaries' whenever financially possible.[70] This was said to be a 'largely negative programme' compared to the 'positive ideals' espoused by COS founder, Sir Charles Loch, when he suggested to a House of Lords Select Committee four years earlier that hospitals should appoint some form of 'charitable assessor, or co-operator ... well instructed as to all forms of relief other than medical'.[71] However, the profession quickly adopted this financial focus. Even before the First World War, both the Hospital Almoners Committee (the national association of almoners) and the Hospital Almoners' Council (which dealt with training and qualifications) had placed tackling 'abuse' at the heart of their definitions of the role.[72]

Once hospitals had appointed almoners in order to serve this financial role, the almoners themselves pushed for a move towards a greater emphasis on social work. For example, Alan Moncrieff, Nuffield Professor of Child Health at the University of London, wrote in 1948 that in the half-century since the appointment of the first almoner:

> medical-social work has moved away from the narrow conception of negatively preventing abuse of the hospital's charity towards the positive aspect of contributing to the diagnosis and treatment of disease by providing the medical staff with details of the social background against which the patients' symptoms must be judged, and his or her treatment adjusted.[73]

This finance-first narrative fits the case of Bristol, where almoners were introduced with a clear focus on recovering payment over social work. The appointment of the city's first almoners came alongside the 1921 introduction of a payment scheme. Similarly, almoners began to be appointed in public hospitals – beginning with Surrey and London – only in the 1930s, when 'appropriated' municipal hospitals had a duty to recover their costs from patients where possible.[74]

Whether the financial side or social work is said to have come first, the professional literature was agreed on the eventual primacy of the social work aspect. This was perhaps most forcefully asserted by Flora Beck, a social worker and social work scholar attached to the Nuffield Department of Medicine:

The almoner is a social worker in a medical setting, and medical social work differs from other forms of social work only in this, that its particular concern with social problems is in relation to health and sickness. Social case work has been defined in this context as 'the art of helping people, both through the best use of their own capabilities and through the resources of the community, to overcome personal and social difficulties, and to achieve the fullest possible measure of health and independence'.[75]

A similar view was expressed in a mid-1930s report of the almoner's department at Addenbrooke's Hospital in Cambridge, which makes no mention of payment whatsoever:

Each Department of the Hospital sees the patient from a different angle. In the Almoner's Office he is no longer the gangrenous appendix, the obstinate arthritis, or the glaucoma that has responded so well to treatment, but an ordinary human being with his background of ordinary human cares and relationships. He is for us the out-of-work trying to balance a budget that can never quite meet the household needs; an Old Age Pensioner without kith or kin; a child whose future still hangs precariously in the balance. Through the Almoner's Office pass all the types which go to make up the Hospital world, the lonely, the misfits, the discouraged and the difficult – all through sickness or poverty, in need of some help or advice.[76]

It is certainly true that assessment for financial purposes was only one of many jobs carried out by the almoner. In some unusual cases, alternative arrangements relieved them of this responsibility altogether. For example, at King's College Hospital: 'If you didn't produce your voucher, or the promise of it, you put something in a box. You kind of bought a ticket and so the medical social workers there didn't have any responsibility for assessment.'[77] Even where they did conduct financial assessments they might not always be the top priority. One former almoner recalled her attitude years later, which she found an easier fit with working in a London County Council institution, rather than a voluntary hospital: 'If I've got several people outside my door in outpatients with difficult problems, and others are just waiting for me to assess whether they can manage one and sixpence per attendance or not, there is no question in my mind where I'm going to spend the time.'[78] This became easier still during the Second World War, which another almoner remembered as 'a great opportunity, because the emergency medical service which was a trial run for the National Health Service, put an end to all these patients' payments and things. The contributory schemes kept on, but they took care of so much that gradually the almoners were able to get out of that administrative chore.'[79]

Beyond financial assessments almoners took on a wide range of roles more easily understood as 'social work'. These included giving advice on hospital procedures, public benefits and how to make medically necessary changes at home and work. They arranged transfers to other institutions, including admission to a convalescent home, established rehabilitation plans and organised after-care visitations. It fell to them to find emergency accommodation for patients' relatives when they were admitted and ensure that family and community networks of support were in place when they were discharged. They might also act as a patient's advocate to secure public or voluntary services, such as funded admission to an appropriate special school for a sick child. The task was theirs of making practical arrangements for surgical appliances, such as artificial limbs or hearing aids. The professional literature said it was also their job to deal with 'misfits', including 'employable cripples' and the 'mentally handicapped'.[80] In this role, the almoner therefore served 'as a link between the medical and social worlds and to see the patient not merely as a "case" but as a distinctive personality'.[81] As this involved directing patients to support from both public and voluntary sources, the almoner profession has been said to embody the 'inter-weaving of statutory and voluntary service' historically characteristic of the British welfare system, operating at the hub of its mixed economy.[82]

In Bristol, the almoner's focus was on assessments for the payment scheme and the financial side of the role, even if they might have wished otherwise. This was demonstrated, for example, by the Bristol Homeo-pathic Hospital judging the almoner's work in 1937 to have been satis-factory due to the continued increase in the number of patients 'who are members of Contributory or Works Medical Charity Schemes'.[83] Similarly, the appointment of a second Assistant Almoner was 'justified' on the grounds that it would generate 'a still further rise in income, and in an increase of general efficiency'.[84] Meanwhile 'after-care' work was given a 'comparatively small amount of time'.[85] Across Bristol's hospitals this was a secondary aspect of the role, but not an entirely overlooked one. The substantial work of almoners in securing continued support after discharge was an important contribution to the integration of local care services across the mixed economy of welfare.[86]

'Very frequently the best and most useful social work consists not in any material form of help,' the Bristol Royal Infirmary's almoner noted in 1922, 'but in the establishment of the friendly relation with the patient, which makes it possible to give advice and guidance of real value.'[87] To this end, 'home visits' also featured as part of the almoner's after-care work in her reports.[88] By the late 1920s, the practice had developed whereby subscribers to convalescent homes would send their recommendation tickets to her for use in the after-care referral of hospital patients.[89] In this respect, she was part of the wider network of voluntary healthcare and charitable institutions. This was also seen in 1931, when 'a grant was made from Clifton College Chapel Sick and Poor Fund to be used at the Almoner's discretion for needy patients'.[90] She was also engaged with voluntary efforts at the hospital itself; for example in encouraging the establishment of a Samaritan Fund to support the non-medical needs of patients, eventually set up at the Bristol Royal Infirmary in 1938, a decade after that of the Bristol General Hospital.[91] The department would also commonly organise free rail travel, or the lending of a motor car for transporting patients unable to travel by bus or train, to hospital or convalescent homes: 'The patients themselves constantly affirm that to be taken to Weston or Clevedon by car is the "best bit" of the Convalescence!'[92] Comments in the almoner's report for the Infirmary in 1937 suggest the department was involved in road accident cases, both providing grants until insurance claims might be resolved but also gathering evidence to support those claims.[93]

The close working relationship between the almoner's department and charitable organisations outside the hospital, as well as the traditional charitable subscribers to the hospital, emerges in the very first almoner's report for a Bristol hospital:

A.B., a girl of 14 years, was in the Women's Medical Ward suffering from acute Chorea. It was not the first attack and during her short life she had been several times in the Infirmary. The child's father was an invalid and as the mother had to go out to work, there was no one to look after the patient after her return home. She was quite unfit to work and would have been left to her own devices all day long. By the doctor's advice the Almoner sent A.B. for two months to the Herbert Home at

Bournemouth. It was necessary to obtain four subscriber's 'letters' which reduced the weekly charge to 9s. 6. The Civic League made enquiries into the case and raised the necessary money, the child's mother paying part of the weekly charge, A.B. returned from Bournemouth very much improved in health and the doctor pronounced her fit for work.

A light place has been found for her in service and she is being kept under Medical observation from the Infirmary.[94]

Almoning as a career

Clearly the almoner was an important figure in the voluntary hospital, yet we know little about who became almoners or their career paths. We do know the almoner profession was a 'predominantly female' one in contrast to the typically male enquiry officers who preceded them.[95] Indeed, the case of Thomas William Cramp, Outpatient Inspector from the 1890s turned almoner at the Metropolitan Hospital in London between 1902 and 1923, was a rare occurrence and merited special attention in posterity.[96] Given the notable involvement in the domestic arrangements of patients we can place the almoner firmly within the 'feminine public sphere', able to draw upon the moral authority of the middle-class woman over working-class motherhood and domestic-ity.[97] Yet at the same time, amongst female careers, the position of almoner conferred both high status and reasonably high pay.

Before the First World War, an almoner's salary was advertised as between £100 and £200 per year, up to ten times that for general domestic servant at the time.[98] In the 1930s, starting salaries were often three times those of nurses.[99] Almoning was a career for educated women, but it was not amongst the best paid, with higher salaries available in education and the Civil Service. Graduate female teachers in secondary schools earned £359 a year on average in 1923, while the few women in senior administrative Civil Service posts a decade later earned more than £700 a year.[100] Yet such salaries were far from the norm for working women. In her 1935 advice for women seeking careers, feminist Ray Strachey wrote that 'At present wages range, roughly speaking, from £1 to £4 a week, and salaries from £3 to £5; and the numbers of women workers who earn more than this are inconsid-erable' and '£250 a year is quite an achievement, even for a highly quali-fied woman with years of experience.'[101] While she described social work as a career 'undertaken in a vocational spirit', with salaries of around £150 'not good', almoners' salaries were higher, typically between £200 and £300.[102] By 1942, the Institute of Hospital Almoners was recommending almoners be paid a yearly salary according to the following scale:

Head Almoner with assistants	£350–£500 per annum
Single-handed Almoner	£250–£350
Assistant Almoner with experience	£225 minimum
Assistant Almoner in first post	£200 rising to £250 over four years [103]

This level of pay required significant training. In Bristol this involved two years' study at university as well as placements with hospitals and the Council of Social Service. In the late 1930s, the Bristol Royal Infirmary's almoner described the role of their students:

> We have two or three students each term who are studying for their Social Study Diploma, and they are able to concentrate on visits to the patients' homes; in this way it is possible to keep in touch with many patients requiring assistance with Housing conditions, advice on difficult diets, to say nothing of the number of problems surrounding those who are discharged before they are fully able to take up their normal livelihood again. In return these students obtain valuable experience, and contacts with different aspects of Hospital life and administration. In addition to the University students the Institute of Hospital Almoners send students for their one or two months' Provincial training during which time they are able to see the full work of the department.[104]

In fact, the University of Bristol was one of only thirteen institutions where these necessary courses could be taken. Three of the others were in London: Bedford College, King's College of Household and Social Science and the London School of Economics. The only others in the provincial south were Oxford School of Social Study and Southampton University College (until 1939). The others were Leeds, Liverpool, Birmingham, Manchester, Nottingham, Edinburgh and Glasgow Universities.[105] As such, Bristol was a regional centre in the development of the almoner profession just as much as it was for medical services. Consequently, the almoner profession may well have been more developed or better supported in Bristol than in some other cities.

Having undertaken this training, almoners played what was widely understood to be an important social role. As Jane Lewis commented, the almoner 'was perceived as the person responsible for forging the crucial links between individual, family and community, and hence to the wider society and state'.[106] Indeed, in the almoner profession we can see women 'able to exercise considerable influence on the direction of social provision' at the point of delivery.[107] Taking on such a role was in turn an implicitly political act, fitting as it did the description of 'useful public service' that was one of the four demands set out in a *Labour Women* editorial in 1922 calling for greater political engagement.[108]

Almoners and patients

The first point of contact between the almoner and the patient would take place in her office for outpatients, as shown in figure 3.4, and usually on the ward for inpatients.[109] One professional guide described the task:

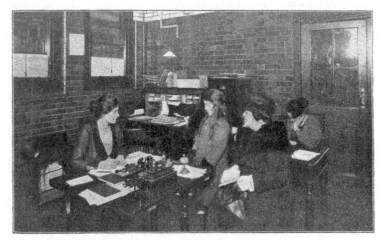

THE ALMONER OF THE GREAT NORTHERN HOSPITAL AT WORK.

Figure 3.4 Almoner interviewing patients in London hospital, *c.*1920

> At her first interview with a patient, the almoner has two important
> things to do. The first is to determine whether social problems are likely
> to have a bearing on the patient's illness. The second is to make the
> patient feel that here is a person with whom he could, if necessary,
> discuss his personal difficulties; someone to whom he need not mind
> admitting any trivial misunderstanding which had been bothering him,
> and to whom he could reveal serious and confidential problems without
> embarrassment.[110]

During this interview, the almoner would endeavour to establish 'the
income and the chief items of expenditure of a family, the type of work
on which its members are engaged, and later on such salient facts as
their religion and amusements, as well as the characteristics of the
home'. This could then be followed up by further investigation, where
necessary and with the patient's agreement, by seeking information 'not
only from the patient, but also through other social agencies, from relatives, from employers, or from other sources'; and with inpatients 'by
consultation with the sister of the ward'.[111] In the professional literature
it was said to be a 'golden rule' that this should take place after the
patient had seen the doctor, so that admission should be a medical
matter and such financial considerations secondary.[112] What is less
clear is whether this distinction had any meaning for the patients
themselves.

Although in the professional debates of the day much was made of
the tension between these social and financial roles of the almoner,
there was in practice something of a natural fit between them. Beck gave
two reasons for the almoner's practice of 'social enquiry' into the personal circumstances of the patient. They were, first, 'to discover whether
social factors such as poverty, bad housing, unsuitable working conditions, or personal worries and maladjustments may have affected the
illness'; and, second, 'to get as complete a picture of the personal, social
and economic background as may be necessary when social assistance
is required'.[113] An omitted third was that it informed the level at which
a financial contribution would be requested. As Manchée noted, it was
because the almoner was approaching the patient holistically that she
was seen as being most capable of making these investigations and
judging the individual's ability to pay in a 'fair' way.[114]

Indeed, when in December 1935 the Glasgow Royal Infirmary
introduced 'a three month experiment empowering the almoners to

encourage patients who could afford it to contribute something towards their maintenance', they believed the almoner could administer such a scheme 'in a kindly and judicious manner without giving the slightest cause for resentment on the part of any patient'.[115] Beck similarly described the relationship between the almoner and the patient as a cordial one, realistically responding to changing times:

> Since almoners first started their work the function of the hospitals has itself changed; what used primarily to be charities dispensing free medical treatment to those who could not afford a general practitioner's fee have gradually been transformed into centres for specialist treatment which could not be obtained outside. The relationship between patient and hospital has changed accordingly, and in recent years the majority of patients have been anxious to make sure that the hospital received payment from a contributory scheme or some other source, or else themselves to pay on a business-like footing for services received. [116]

The evidence is mixed on whether or not patients perceived this to be the 'fair' system described by practitioners. While Steven Cherry has suggested that almoners 'were often resented', the few surviving accounts display a wider range of responses.[117] One woman, born in 1930, has recalled: 'An august but very kind lady called the Lady Almoner would come round the wards and inquire as to a patient's financial resources. If you could you would make a contribution. If not, there was no pressure or feelings of shame. Very benign I remember.'[118] Another, less positive, reference to the almoner can be found in the memoir of Bella Aronovitch, who was moved around a variety of London hospitals in the late 1920s when suffering with appendicitis. She recalled:

> A few days after this first operation I had a visit from the hospital almoner. She came into the ward carrying a huge sheaf of papers and looked terrifyingly efficient. Following a few minutes' talk with Sister she came over to me, made herself comfortable on a chair beside my bed and for the next quarter of an hour, her conversation consisted entirely of questions. She started with questions about my family. How many of us were at home? Who went to work and who were still at school? How much did I earn when I went to work? How much rent did we pay? What was our total income from all sources? etc., etc. Now all the questions were the preliminary skirmishes to the final question, which was; could my family afford to pay towards my upkeep while I was in hospital and if so,

how much? ... I found all those questions rather trying. However, I answered them as truthfully and to the best of my ability. As the almoner left, she told me to be sure to tell my mother to call at her office next mid-week visiting day. She then double checked with Mother on the answers to all questions.[119]

Falling somewhere between those accounts, and echoing the idea that payment was not explicitly optional, an oral history project conducted into health services in Lancashire suggests that there was some understanding of the non-compulsory nature of such systems. Mrs Carson (born in 1902) recounted outpatients being treated free and inpatients being sent 'a bill': 'They didn't force you to pay it, but they would ask you to pay something or make a donation to the hospital if [you] couldn't afford to pay the bill, with more or less everybody paying something.' When scalded at work she ended up spending her twenty-first birthday at Lancaster Infirmary. She recalled: 'I got a bill for it. Six bob a day.'[120] More critically, in an article celebrating the sixtieth anniversary of the NHS, one trade unionist wrote the following:

> During the second world war a woman is discharged from a south London hospital. Before she leaves the building with her young son they must see the Lady Almoner, who will determine the fees she must pay for her treatment and medicine.
>
> The Lady Almoner sits behind a large wooden desk. She quizzes the woman about her household finances, the income and savings of everyone in the family and their daily standard of living. The interrogation over, the woman takes out her purse, pays the sum demanded, and leaves.
>
> It is an upsetting and humiliating experience for my mother. For me, it is an early introduction to the world of means testing.[121]

There is, therefore, a significant diversity of experiences of the almoner among the few recorded. A similar range is suggested locally by comments that 'In almost every case the patients have been very ready to pay what they could afford' alongside long-running complaints about the misconception of compulsory fees.[122] These varied reactions and recollections suggest that patient responses to the almoner 'ranged from deferential gratitude to pragmatic acceptance to outright resentment', just as Martin Gorsky has noted for recipient responses to Victorian philanthropy.[123] Indeed, we should understand the experience of being assessed by the almoner as a philanthropic encounter.

Hospital contributory schemes

Just as there was confusion over almoner-assessed payment, commonly mistaken for compulsory charges, there was confusion over what benefits could be purchased by membership of a hospital contributory scheme. It was not unusual to join a scheme in order to secure a form of social insurance, and this was something greatly encouraged in the promotion of the schemes (discussed further in chapter 5). The contributory schemes, however, did not provide medical insurance. Strictly speaking, members did not have any additional right of access. The British Hospitals Contributory Scheme made it plainly clear that a contributory scheme: 'Is not an Insurance Scheme, but is a Voluntary Organisation'. Membership, they insisted, 'cannot give any right to contributors to admission to any Hospital, nor any priority right in regard to order of admission', which they said were 'medical questions outside the scope of a Contributory Scheme'.

> The privileges of the Scheme in regard to Hospitals commence to operate *after* the patient has been admitted to Hospital for treatment, and should be limited to securing for the Contributor immunity from any payment towards cost of maintenance in Hospital. Where the privileges of the Fund are based on income limits, the Contributory Scheme should also secure the Contributor immunity from questions in regard to his or her circumstances.[124]

Rather than insurance, therefore, we should understand contributory schemes as part of a tradition of hospital fundraising. Indeed, they were not the first efforts designed to encourage donations and contributions from the working classes. Hospital Sunday was introduced locally to raise funds for the Bristol Royal Infirmary and the Bristol General Hospital in 1860.[125] By the First World War, works governors committees had become more common. By these means, local workpeople donating were represented on the management boards of the Bristol Royal Infirmary, the Bristol General Hospital and Cossham Memorial Hospital.[126] Other typical forms of donation included collection boxes, which were especially promoted by one Bristol contributory scheme in the 1930s. Working-class attitudes towards collection boxes may, in some cases, have mirrored those expressed in the Edwardian novel *The Ragged Trousered Philanthropists*, which sought to document working-class life:

On the ledge of the little window through which their [wages were] passed there was always a Hospital collection-box. Every man put either a penny or twopence into this box. Of course, it was not compulsory to do so, but they all did, because they felt that any man who omitted to contribute might be 'marked'. They did not all agree with contributing to the Hospital, for several reasons. They knew the doctors at the Hospital made a practice of using the free patients to make experiments upon, and they also knew that the so-called 'free' patients who contribute so very largely directly to the maintenance of such institutions, get scant consideration when they apply for 'free' treatment, and are plainly given to understand that they are receiving 'charity'. Some of the men thought that, considering the extent to which they contributed, they should be entitled to attention as a right.[127]

Contributory schemes in Bristol

Once payment schemes were introduced as a means of eliciting a financial contribution from patients, questions were raised about those who had already contributed in response to these fundraising efforts. There was, at least in theory, a standing arrangement at the Bristol Royal Infirmary, in a by-law dating from the appointment of the almoner, that 'where previous arrangements have been made for the contributions payable, no enquiry shall be made'.[128] This would allow for treatment free at the point of need for all those who had subscribed to a workplace fund. Despite this, it appears the medical faculty were committed to the notion that the only distinctions between patients should be medical ones.[129] They insisted it was a matter of principle that 'preferential treatment is not given to any patients', regardless of protestations from the local contributing firm, J.S. Fry and Sons, that 'some scheme should be devised whereby those who contribute to the Infirmary Funds should have priority over those who make no contribution'.[130]

The momentum for a change in the hospital's position appears to have built up during the middle of the decade, while the governors were considering the development of a public contributory scheme along the lines of the pioneering Sheffield penny-in-the-pound scheme, which had been established in 1922.[131] Representatives of various Bristol hospitals met in 1926 to discuss establishing a city-wide contributory scheme. The objectives of the scheme were planned to be 'the raising of Funds for the upkeep of all Institutions of the list, and on behalf of those entitled to benefit, making provisions for the whole or part payment of the charges for maintenance at the same'; whereas admission would be determined by the hospitals, considering only 'the necessity of the case'. Any question of payment would thereafter be a separate consideration.[132] When the BMICS was established a year later, however, it developed along lines quite different, leading the hospitals to set up the BHF as their own rival scheme after twelve years of disagreement on a number of issues. One was whether it was preferable to collaborate with the great number of independent local and workplace schemes, each setting their own rate of subscription, or to unify contributory effort in the city. The BMICS saw itself as working with the smaller schemes and for its members, who had majority control on its governing committee, whereas the BHF worked hard to amalgamate the independent schemes and bring them under the direction of the hospitals. For the BHF, therefore, the proper role of the contributory scheme was more simply as a fundraising adjunct of the hospital.[133]

Despite tensions between the two schemes, there was in fact a degree of unspoken consensus on the question of the range of services to be provided. In 1935, the BMICS set up an Extended Benefits Scheme, which offered cash benefits to contributors when they were admitted to hospital, as well as additional surgical services or convalescent home care.[134] The BMICS was proud that this new scheme was 'the first of its kind in the United Kingdom', and it has been considered a pioneer by historians (since most contributory schemes in the 1950s operated cash grants schemes).[135] However, in the 1930s the scheme's focus on providing financial support to patient-members rather than the hospitals was controversial, with the BMICS called upon to justify it at annual general meetings of the British Hospital Contributory Schemes Association in both 1936 and 1937. In doing so, the BMICS's founding Honorary Secretary, Mr J.S. Tudor 'maintained that this matter was entirely outside the province of the Contributory Scheme Movement, as the accounts were separated from those of the ordinary Contributory Scheme, and that the Scheme was being managed by a committee which had no jurisdiction of the Committee of the Bristol Medical Institutions Contributory Scheme and vice versa'.[136]

The hospitals were not reassured and became increasingly resentful of this scheme, claiming cash benefits to patients to be 'inimical to the interests of the Voluntary Hospitals' for diverting funds from the general support of the institutions, and this became a key disagreement as the relationship between the BMICS and the voluntary hospitals broke down almost entirely.[137] Indeed, hospital representatives went so far as suggesting changing 'its name to Bristol Welfare Association in order that it is completely dis-associated [sic] in the minds of the public from hospital contributory schemes.'[138] Surprisingly, given the concern of the voluntary hospitals, when the BMICS restricted the Extended Benefits Scheme to its members, the BHF felt 'obliged to create a separate Welfare Fund' for its own members. We might say that outright competition for contributors forged a local consensus over what services ought to be provided.[139]

Despite this shared trend for increasingly insurance-style services, both remained organisations firmly rooted in the voluntary sector, in line with the image presented by the cover of the BHF's 1945 report (see figure 3.5), which depicted the various insurance-style schemes as contributing to success in fundraising. This was seen in practice when it took over the administration of the charitable Lord Mayor's Fund in 1941, essentially creating a central clearing house for contributory and charitable donations to the city's voluntary hospitals.[140] The rival BMICS had also shown itself to be fundraising for the hospitals when, more than a decade earlier, over 1,000 of its collection boxes appeared within ten miles of the city centre in just its first two years.[141] In addition to this, from 1931 charitable donations from individuals or workpeople's funds could be earmarked for specific institutions, allowing for a traditional philanthropic relationship between the donor and recipient institution to be rolled out to a far broader base of donors.[142] Perhaps most significantly, while the majority of the BMICS's income would always come from employees and individual contributors, its expenditure was not limited to covering patient payments.[143] In fact grants to the hospitals matched payments on behalf of their members, either taking the form of donations for specific causes, such as the Bristol Royal Infirmary's Cancer Research Fund, or general grants for the upkeep of the institution.[144] In neither case can these funds be seen as insurance payments for their members as patients.

Conclusion

Understanding the almoner and the payment system she administered brings greater clarity to our view of hospital contributory schemes.

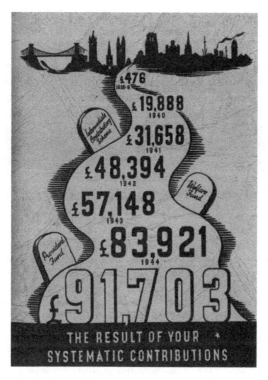

Figure 3.5 Bristol Hospitals Fund schemes depicted as fundraising successes, 1945

The Bristol case suggests the 'consumer choice' generated by reciprocal arrangements between schemes and hospitals, effectively creating a 'voucher' system, that Cherry identified in East Anglia, was far from universal.[145] In the previous chapter we saw how the various hospitals of Bristol covered largely different medical needs. Even when the local authority turned Southmead into a municipal general hospital, it was really only emergency admissions and maternity cases that were taken in Southmead. By contrast, maternity patients already had a choice between numerous voluntary hospitals, often situated nearby each other in the city centre.[146] Bristol provided an urban context for a significant concentration of hospitals operating the same or similar admissions policies. Consequently there was little need for any contributory scheme 'voucher' arrangement to provide choice between institutions.

More fundamentally, as we have seen, admission was not conditional on either almoner-assessed payment or contributory scheme membership. This removes the fundamental premise for seeing them as effectively private healthcare or medical insurance. Instead, both need to be incorporated into our understanding of the medical philanthropy of the voluntary hospital in the early twentieth century. This requires us to recognise that medical philanthropy was not something static. Indeed, the hospital itself was changing at this time and perceptions of the hospital as a charity changed with it. As the city's first almoner wrote in 1921:

> The Bristol Royal Infirmary has been in existence since 1735, as an entirely free Institution and the inhabitants of the City and surrounding district have looked upon it in that light. Charity as represented by voluntary hospitals has become so much part of the established order of things that it is often not regarded as charity at all. It is quite a common occurrence to hear a patient who is receiving free hospital treatment refuse any offer of additional help on the plea that they cannot accept charity.[147]

There were certainly practical changes taking place. However, it is a significant overstatement to view these changes as the end of medical charity. Instead, by offering exemptions from the new payments and maintaining the social encounter that mediated the provision of free hospital care, the almoner was crucial in ensuring these changes amounted to a reinvention, rather than an abandonment, of charitable admission.

The evidence from Bristol's contributory schemes suggests that a working solution was found to balancing fundraising and benefits, although admission was not one of those benefits. Making such fine balances (mis)understood was, however, another matter altogether, and one to which we will return in chapter 5. Whatever the motivation behind membership, hospital contributory schemes were essentially fundraising bodies. Their activities included raising funds for particular campaigns and in some cases grants for the general upkeep of hospitals. Even in their primary function of covering working-class patients' payments they were not playing any role in securing access; rather, they were facilitating voluntary financial contributions on the part of the local population. Where admission was a medical matter, the almoner and the contributory scheme both served to negotiate the terms of that admission. It is in this way that they both played a part in operating a new, but still philanthropic, patient contract in the general wards of the hospitals until 1948.

Notes

1 Sir Alan Garrett Anderson, HC Deb 8 May 1936, vol. 311, c. 2052
2 See especially Steven Cherry, 'Accountability, Entitlement, and Control Issues and Voluntary Hospital Funding c1860–1939', *Social History of Medicine*, 9:2 (1996), 215; Martin Gorsky, *Patterns of Philanthropy: Charity and Society in Nineteenth-Century Bristol* (Woodbridge: Boydell & Brewer Ltd, 1999), pp. 121 and 189.
3 Mary Fissell, 'Charity Universal? Institutions and Moral Reform in Eighteenth-Century Bristol' in Lee Davison, Tim Hitchcock, Tim Keirn and Robert Shoemaker (eds), *Still The Grumbling Hive: The Response to Social and Economic Problems in England, 1689–1750* (Stroud: St Martin's Press, 1992), p. 126; Mary Fissell, *Patients, Power, and the Poor in Eighteenth-Century Bristol* (Cambridge: Cambridge University Press, 1991), p. 7.
4 Fissell, *Patients, Power, and the Poor*, p. 7.
5 Fissell, 'Charity Universal?', p. 121.
6 Fissell, *Patients, Power, and the Poor*, pp. 74 and 12.
7 Alan Kidd, 'Philanthropy and the "Social History Paradigm"', *Social History*, 2:2 (1996), 138; Gorsky, *Patterns of Philanthropy*, p. 121.
8 Elizabeth Gaskell, *Mary Barton: A Tale of Manchester Life*, 2003 Penguin Classics edition (1848), p. 70.
9 Sanctuary, Association of Hospital Officers Conference, 1925, in *Gazette*, May 1925, p. 9, cited in Cherry, 'Accountability', p. 224.
10 This system was also widely used in the United States. See Paul Starr, *The Social Transformation of American Medicine* (New York: Basic Books, 1982), p. 153.
11 Gorsky, *Patterns of Philanthropy*, p. 189.
12 C Bruce Perry, *Voluntary Medical Institutions* (Bristol: Bristol Branch of the Historical Association, 1984), p. 15.
13 Royal Free Hospital Archive, RFH/1/2/2, 'History of the Royal Free Hospital', Royal Free Hospital Reports 1848–65, Book A1, Royal Free Hospital Report, January 1849, p. vii cited in Lynsey Cullen, 'The First Lady Almoner: The Appointment, Position, and Findings of Miss Mary Stewart at the Royal Free Hospital, 1895–99', *Journal of the History of Medicine and Allied Sciences* 68:4 (2013), 559 (original emphasis).

14 Martin Gorsky, John Mohan, and Martin Powell, 'The Financial Health of Voluntary Hospitals in Interwar Britain', *Economic History Review*, 55:3 (2002), 476; Martin Daunton, 'Payment and Participation: Welfare and State-Formation in Britain, 1990–1951', *Past and Present*, 150 (1990), 188–91.

15 Radcliffe Infirmary, *Report* (1919), p. 11; Centre for Oxfordshire Studies, OXFO 362.1 RADC, 'Letter Explaining the Abolition of the "Turns" System at the Radcliffe Infirmary', June 1926.

16 Nick Hayes, '"Our Hospitals"? Voluntary Provision, Community and Civic Consciousness in Nottingham Before the NHS', *Midland History*, 37:1 (2012), 98–9.

17 Jonathan Reinarz, *Health Care in Birmingham: The Birmingham Teaching Hospitals, 1779–1939* (Woodbridge: Boydell Press, 2014).

18 See especially Steven Cherry, 'Beyond National Health Insurance. The Voluntary Hospitals and Hospital Contributory Schemes: A Regional Study', *Social History of Medicine*, 5:3 (1992), 455–82; Cherry, 'Accountability'; Steven Cherry, 'Before the National Health Service: Financing the Voluntary Hospitals, 1900–1939', *Economic History Review*, 50:2 (1997), 305–26; Steven Cherry, 'Hospital Saturday, Workplace Collections and Issues in Late Nineteenth-Century Hospital Funding', *Medical History*, 44:4 (2000), 461–88; Martin Gorsky, John Mohan and Tim Willis, 'Hospital Contributory Schemes and the NHS Debates 1937–46: The Rejection of Social Insurance in the British Welfare State?', *Twentieth Century British History*, 16:2 (2005), 170–92; Martin Gorsky, John Mohan and Tim Willis, 'From Hospital Contributory Schemes to Health Cash Plans: The Mutual Ideal in British Health Care after 1948', *Journal of Social Policy*, 34:3 (2005), 447–67; Martin Gorsky, John Mohan, with Tim Willis, *Mutualism and Health Care: British Hospital Contributory Schemes in the Twentieth Century* (Manchester: Manchester University Press, 2006); Barry M. Doyle, 'Power and Accountability in the Voluntary Hospitals of Middlesbrough 1900–48' in Peter Shapely and Anne Borsay (ed.), *Medicine, Charity and Mutual Aid: The Consumption of Health and Welfare, c.1550–1950* (Aldershot: Ashgate, 2006), pp. 207–24; Barry M. Doyle, 'Competition and Cooperation in Hospital Provision in Middlesbrough, 1918–1948', *Medical History*, 51:3 (2007), 337–56; Barry M. Doyle, 'Labour and Hospitals in Three Yorkshire Towns: Middlesbrough, Leeds, Sheffield, 1919–1938', *Social History of Medicine*, 23:2 (2010), 374–92.

19 Gorsky and Mohan, *Mutualism and Health Care*, p. 64; Cherry, 'Beyond', p. 455.

20 Gorsky and Mohan, *Mutualism*, p. 49.

21 *Bristol Times and Mirror*, 2 July 1921, p. 7.

22 Charles Saunders, *The Bristol Eye Hospital* (Bristol: United Bristol Hospitals, 1960), p. 24; V.J. Marmion, *The Bristol Eye Hospital: A Monograph* (Bristol, 1987), p. 18; Bristol Homeopathic Hospital, *Report for 1937*, pp. 25–6.

23 Reinarz, 'Investigating the "Deserving" Poor'.

24 Bristol Children's Hospital, *Report for 1920*, p. 5.

25 Bristol Children's Hospital, *Report for 1921*, pp. 20 and 12; Charles Saunders, *The Bristol Royal Hospital for Sick Children* (Bristol: United Bristol Hospitals, 1961), p.20. A similar issue was noted in nineteenth-century Birmingham in Reinarz, 'Investigating the "Deserving" Poor'.

26 Cherry, 'Insurance', pp. 467 and 464.

27 Bristol Homeopathic Hospital, *Report for 1937*, p. 5.

28 Mark Abrams, *The Conditions of the British People, 1911–1945* (London: Victor Gollancz, 1946), pp. 84–5.

29 Ministry of Labour, *Eighteenth Abstract of Labour Statistics of the United Kingdom* (London: HMSO, 1926), pp. 104–7.

30 'Minutes of Meeting of Joint Sub-Committee of Bristol Royal Infirmary and Bristol General Hospital on the subject of Paying Patients held at Exchange Chambers, Bristol, on Tuesday, April 10th 1921 at 5pm', in BRI, Faculty Minutes 1911–1925, p. 241.

31 BRI, *Report for 1926*, p. 19.

32 BRI, *Report for 1921*, p. 10

33 BRI, *Report for 1922*, p. 21.

34 *Ibid.*, p. 19.

35 *Bristol Times and Mirror*, 2 July 1921, p. 7.

36 Bristol Homeopathic Hospital, *Report for 1937*, pp. 25–6.

37 BRI, *Report for 1923*, p. 21.

38 Cherry, 'Accountability', p. 230.

39 BRI, *Report for 1922*, p. 21 and *Report for 1932*, p. 18; BGH, *Report for 1933*, p. 21.

40 University of Nottingham Library, Manuscripts Department, UHe M1/7, Mins Finance and House Comm., Eye Hospital, 12 June and 10 July 1912; Uhg M/1/4, Report of the Almoner, General Hospital, 6 Oct. 1937, cited in Hayes, 'Our Hospitals?', p. 101.

41 Hayes, 'Our Hospitals?', p. 101.

42 BRI, *Report 1921*, p. 20. In 1938, the same promise, that nobody had ever been refused treatment from an inability to pay, was be made by the Secretary of the Nottingham General Hospital. See Hayes 'Our Hospitals?', p. 98.

43 BRI, House Committee Minutes, 6 January 1925.

44 John Stewart, '"The Finest Municipal Hospital Service in the World"?: Contemporary Perceptions of the London County Council's Hospital Provision, 1929–1939', *Urban History*, 32:2 (2005), 327–44.

45 Parsons, 'Bristol', p. 142.

46 BCM, 1 January 1930.

47 Barry M. Doyle, *A History of Hospitals in Middlesbrough* (Middlesbrough: South Tees NHS Hospitals Trust, 2003), p. 62.

48 Barry M. Doyle, *The Politics of Hospital Provision in Early 20th-Century Britain* (London: Pickering and Chatto, 2014), p. 64.

49 BCM, 1 January 1930.

50 BCM, 10 October 1933, Report of the Health Committee, 26 September 1933.

51 Almoner's Report, Southmead Hospital, in BMOH, *Report for 1937*, p. 156.

52 Lara Marks, *Metropolitan Maternity: Maternal and Infant Welfare Service in Early Twentieth Century London* (Amsterdam: Rodopi, 1996).

53 BRI, Faculty Minutes, 20 November 1919; Bristol Children's Hospital, *Report for 1920*, pp. 11–12.

54 *Ibid.*, Faculty Minutes, 20 July 1918; General Committee Minutes, 23 July 1918.

55 *Ibid.*, General Committee Minutes, 13 January 1920.

56 Bruce Perry, *Voluntary Medical Institutions*, p. 6; Charles Saunders, *The United Bristol Hospitals* (Bristol: United Bristol Hospitals, 1965), p. 63.

57 *Ibid.*, General Committee Minutes, 11 November 1919.

58 *Ibid.*, General Committee Minutes, 9 November 1920.

59 *Bristol Times and Mirror*, 2 July 1921, p. 7.

60 Hayes, 'Our Hospitals?', pp. 98–9.

61 Angela Simmons, *A Profession and Its Roots – The Lady Almoners* (Michelangelo Press, 2005), https://www.kcl.ac.uk/sspp/policy-institute/scwru/swhn/publications/Simmons-A-Profession-and-Its-Roots-The-Lady-Almoners.pdf, accessed 25 April 2016. Similarly, see E. Moberly Bell, *The Story of Hospital Almoners: The Birth of a Profession* (London: Faber & Faber, 1961).

62 Phyllis Willmott, '1895–1945: The First 50 Years' in Joan Baraclough, Grace Dedman, Hazel Osborn and Phyllis Willmott (eds), *100 Years of Health Related Social Work 1895–1995: Then – Now – Onwards* (Birmingham: BASW, 1996), pp. 1–11.

63 Keir Waddington, 'Unsuitable Cases: The Debate over Outpatient Admissions, the Medical Profession and Late-Victorian London Hospitals', *Medical History*, 42:1 (1998), 42–5.

64 See Cullen, 'First Lady Almoner'.

65 Chris Nottingham and Rona Dougall, 'A Close and Practical Association with the Medical Profession: Scottish Medical Social Workers and the Social Medicine, 1940–1975', *Medical History*, 51:3 (2007), 309–36.

66 Elaine Thomson, 'Between Separate Spheres: Medical Women, Moral Hygiene and the Edinburgh Hospital for Women and Children' in Steve Sturdy (ed.), *Medicine, Health and the Public Sphere in Britain 1600–2000* (London, 2002), pp. 116–17.

67 Doyle, *Politics of Hospital Provision*, pp. 70–1.

68 Dorothy Manchée, *Whatever Does the Almoner Do?* (London: Bailliere, Tindall and Cox., 1946), preface.

69 *Ibid.*, pp. 8–9.

70 I.F. Beck, *The Almoner: A Brief Account of Medical Social Service in Great Britain* (London: Council of the Institute of Almoners, 1948), p. 50; *The Hospital Almoner: A Brief Study of Hospital Social Service in Great Britain* (London: Hospital Almoners Association, 1935), p. 39. For an in-depth consideration of Mary Stewart's role as the first hospital almoner see Cullen, 'Almoner'.

71 Beck, *Almoner*, pp. 49–50; *Almoner: Brief Study*, p. 34.

72 Willmott, '50 Years', pp. 3–5.

73 Alan Moncrieff, 'Preface' in Beck, *Almoner*, p. 3.

74 Willmott, '50 Years', p. 7.

75 Beck, *Almoner*, p. 4.

76 Almoner's Report in the Addenbrooke's Hospital, Cambridge, *Report for 1934–1935*, p. 18.

77 Elizabeth Gloyne, Social Workers Speak Out, 1981, 8, Modern Records Centre [hereafter MRC], University of Warwick, http://www2.warwick.ac.uk/services/library/mrc/explorefurther/speakingarchives/social-work/929.publ_no_9_gloyne.pdf, accessed 11 March 2016.

78 Enid Warren, Social Workers Speak Out, 1981, 13, MRC, University of Warwick, http://www2.warwick.ac.uk/services/library/mrc/explorefurther/speakingarchives/socialwork/929.publ_no_21_warren.pdf, accessed 11 March 2016.

79 Jean Snelling, Social Workers Speak Out, 1980, 21, MRC, University of Warwick, http://www2.warwick.ac.uk/services/library/mrc/explore-further/speakingarchives/socialwork/929.publ_no_18_j_snelling.pdf, accessed 11 March 2016.

80 Beck, *Almoner*, pp. 6–7, 10–11, 17–18 and 43; *Almoner: Brief Study*, pp. 55–67; D.A. Dow, M.M. Leitch and A.F. MacLean, *From Almoner to Social Worker: Social Work at Glasgow Royal Infirmary, 1932–1982* (Glasgow: Glasgow Royal Infirmary, 1982), p. 10.

81 Dow, *et al.*, *Social Worker*, p. 9.

82 Marjorie McInnes, 'Preface' in Dow, et al., Social Worker, p. 4.

83 BHH, Report for 1937, p. 25.

84 BRI, Report for 1935, p. 20.

85 BRI, Report for 1921, p. 20.

86 This was noted for Bristol in Gorsky, 'Bristol's Hospital Services', ch. 5.1. See also Martin Gorsky, Martin Powell and John Mohan, 'British Voluntary Hospitals and the Public Sphere: Contribution and Participation before the National Health Service' in Sturdy (ed.), Public Sphere, p. 124.

87 BRI, Report for 1922, pp. 21–2.

88 For example, see BRI, Report for 1924, p. 21.

89 BRI, Report for 1927, p. 17.

90 BRI, Report for 1931, p. 18.

91 BRI, Report for 1936, p. 26; Report for 1938, p. 18; BGH, Report for 1927, p. 20.

92 BRI, Report for 1930, p. 18; Report for 1937, p. 22.

93 BRI, Report for 1937.

94 BRI, Report for 1921, p. 20.

95 Nottingham and Dougall, 'Association', p. 309.

96 Andrew Scakville, 'Thomas William Cramp, Almoner: The Forgotten Man in a Female Profession', British Journal of Social Work, 19:1 (1989), 95–110.

97 For some of the key themes in the literature on women's philanthropic work, see F.K. Prochaska, Women and Philanthropy in Nineteenth-Century England (Oxford: Clarendon Press, 1980); Megan Smitley, The Feminine Public Sphere: Middle-Class Women and Civic Life in Scotland, c.1870–1914 (Manchester: Manchester University Press, 2009); Dorice Williams Elliott, The Angel Out of the House: Philanthropy and Gender in Nineteenth-Century England (London: University of Virginia Press, 2002).

98 A. Frederic White, 'Hospital Almoners' in Every Woman's Encyclopaedia: Articles Relevant to a Woman's Life in Society (London, 1910–1912), http://chestofbooks.com/food/household/Woman-Encyclopaedia-3/Hospital-Almoners.html, accessed 25 April 2016. According to advertisements in The Times the average annual wage for a general servant in 1907 was £19 10s. Elizabeth Roberts, Women's Work, 1840–1940 (Cambridge: Cambridge University Press, 1988), p. 22.

99 Ray Strachey, Careers and Openings for Women: A Survey of Women's Employment and a Guide for Those Seeking Work (London: Faber and Faber, 1935), pp. 223 and 233.

100 Alison Oram, Women Teachers and Feminist Politics, 1900–39 (Manchester: Manchester University Press, 1996), p. 25; Strachey, Careers and Openings, pp. 71–2.

101 Strachey, Careers and Openings, pp. 81 and 70.

102 Ibid., pp. 158–9, 223 and 240.

103 Modern Records Centre [hereafter MRC], Institute of Hospital Almoners [hereafter IHA], *Report for 1942*, p. 10.

104 BRI, *Report for 1937*, p. 21.

105 M, Institute of Hospital Almoners, *Reports for 1938*, p. 17; and *Report for 1939*, p. 15.

106 Jane Lewis, *Women and Social Action in Victorian and Edwardian England* (Stanford: Stanford University Press, 1991), p. 305.

107 Jane Lewis, 'Women, Social Work and Social Welfare in Twentieth-Century Britain: From (Unpaid) Influence to (Paid) Oblivion?' in Martin Daunton (ed.), *Charity, Self-Interest and Welfare in the English Past* (London: UCL Press, 1996), p. 205.

108 Cited in Pat Thane, 'What Difference Did the Vote Make?' in Amanda Vickery (ed.), *Women, Privilege and Power: British Politics, 1750 to the Present* (Stanford: Stanford University Press, 2001), p. 284.

109 Beck, *Almoner: Brief Study*, p. 47.

110 Beck, *The Almoner*, p. 5.

111 Beck, *Almoner*, pp. 8–9; *Almoner: Brief Study*, p. 47.

112 Beck, *Almoner: Brief Study*, p. 41.

113 Beck, *Almoner*, p. 5.

114 Manchée, *Whatever*, p. 9.

115 Dow, *et al.*, *Social Worker*, p. 10.

116 Beck, *Almoner*, p. 60.

117 *Ibid.*, p. 61; Cherry, 'Accountability', p. 230.

118 Rayner Garner, from the UK Midwifery Archives on *Midwifery Matters*, the website of the Association of Radical Midwives, http://www.midwifery.org.uk/?page_id=655, accessed 25 April 2016.

119 Bella Aronovitch, *Give it Time. An Experience of Hospital, 1928–1932* (London: Andre Deutsch, 1974) cited in Deborah Brunton (ed.), *Health, Disease and Society in Europe 1800–1930: A Source Book* (Manchester: Manchester University Press, 2004), p. 285.

120 Lucinda McCray Beier, *For Their Own Good: The Transformation of English Working-Class Health Culture, 1880–1970* (Columbus: Ohio State University Press, 2008), p. 133.

121 Jim Cobley, 'Happy Birthday NHS', TSSA (Transport and Salaried Staffs' Association) Journal, August/September 2008, http://www.tssa.org.uk/article-269.php3?id_article=4349, accessed 9 September 2010.

122 BGH, *Report for 1921*, p. 17; BRI, *Reports for 1921–1938*.

123 Gorsky, *Patterns of Philanthropy*, p. 231.

124 Bristol Contributory Welfare Association [hereafter BCWA], Extracts from British Hospital Contributory Schemes Association Points of Policy

for Hospital Contributory Schemes, 1937 (original emphasis). Gorsky and Mohan acknowledge schemes did not have the 'legal position' of insurance bodies in *Mutualism and Health Care*, p. 65.

125 Bruce Perry, *Voluntary Medical Institutions*, p. 5.

126 See Gorsky and Mohan, *Mutualism and Health Care*, pp. 25–31.

127 Robert Tressell, *The Ragged Trousered Philanthropists* (London: Flamingo Modern Classics edn, 1997 [1914]), p. 221.

128 BSC, Bristol Hospitals Commission, BHF evidence, Representatives, 1926.

129 BRI, Faculty Minutes, 8 December 1919.

130 BRI, House Committee Minutes, 4 September 1919.

131 BRI, General Committee Minutes, 21 April 1925. See Steve Sturdy, 'The Political Economy of Scientific Medicine: Science, Education and the Transformation of Medical Practice in Sheffield, 1890–1922', *Medical History*, 3:6 (1992), 144–5.

132 BSC, DM980 (30), Bristol Hospitals Commission, BHF evidence, appendix 1. 'Report of Meeting of representatives of Bristol Royal Infirmary, Bristol General Hospital and Sub-Committee of Employees to consider the suggested Contributory Scheme' [hereafter Representatives], 30 July 1926.

133 For further details see George Campbell Gosling, ' "Open the Other Eye": Payment, Civic Duty and Hospital Contributory Schemes in Bristol, c.1927–1948', *Medical History*, 54:4 (2010), 475–94.

134 BMICS, *Report for 1934*; Rules adopted, December 1936.

135 BMICS, *Report for 1935*, p. 5; Gorsky and Mohan, *Mutualism and Health Care*, p. 196.

136 BCWA, 'At the 24th Meeting of the Executive Committee of the British Hospitals Contributory Schemes Association', 17 July 1936.

137 BSC, Bristol Hospitals Commission, BHF evidence, 'Communication from the Joint Committee of Hospital Representatives to the Bristol Medical Institutions Contributory Scheme (Inc.)'.

138 BSC, DM980 (28), Contributory Schemes Conference Dinner 1942, Bristol & District Divisional Hospitals Council, schedule 2.

139 BSC, DM980 (35), BHF, 'Summarised Diary of Negotiations to Establish One Central Hospitals Contributory Scheme in Bristol'.

140 BSC, DM980 (12), Lord Mayor's Hospital Fund, Bristol & District Divisional Hospitals Council Sub-Committee, Report of meeting of standing committee sub-committee and the Lord Mayor's Fund sub-committee, 16 November 1942.

141 BMICS, *Report for 1928*, p. 8.

142 BMICS, *Reports for 1931–1945*.

143 BMICS, *Reports for 1928–1945*.
144 BMICS, *Report for 1934*, p. 6; *Report for 1929*, pp. 8–9.
145 Cherry, 'Insurance', p. 475.
146 Cope, *et al.*, *Survey*, pp. 31 and 178.
147 BRI, *Report for 1921*, p. 20.

4

Middle-class medicine

> It is well known that Englishmen are in the main opposed to any and every new system with which they are not familiar. Probably to this influence is due the fact, that, with a few exceptions, pay wards are as unknown in this country as the pay hospitals themselves.[1]
>
> Sir Henry Burdett, founder of the King's Fund, 1879

There was only one area of the pre-NHS hospital system which genuinely saw private healthcare operating on a commercial basis. This was the parallel provision made for middle-class patients, the likes of 'George' from *Your Very Good Health*, in the British hospital of the early twentieth century. Since admission of middle-class patients was commonly seen as a threat to the charitable character of the institution, as will be examined in the next chapter, it became the established practice to have income limits for admission to the ordinary wards. In Bristol these rose from roughly £250 per year in the 1920s to over £400 in the 1940s, roughly in line with the threshold for income tax.[2] Those above this level would have been termed 'middle-class' by the Ministry of Labour and hospital authorities alike, and commonly excluded from accessing hospital services through the mechanisms described in the previous chapter.[3] It was only by charging higher rates to this separate class of patient that the hospitals stood any chance of turning a profit. This new category of patient would be accommodated not in the usual dormitory-style wards, but in a separate one- or occasionally two-bed room, domestic in style. These private wards would be physically separate, sometimes in entirely separate buildings. Charges for such rooms were not voluntary contributions towards the cost of maintenance, but rather compulsory fees set at a rate to cover at least the full cost of treatment. Consequently, where patients in the general wards might pay up to one guinea per week, patients in these private wards could pay up to ten guineas per week. In addition to which they would have to negotiate with the doctor a fee for his services.[4]

Paying the very highest rates was rare, according to confidential briefing papers produced for parliamentarians by the King's Fund, lobbying in support of more voluntary hospital services for private patients. Surveying the provision on offer in London in the mid-1930s, the King's Fund categorised the different rates charged as fitting for patients of 'limited means' (up to three guineas per week), 'moderate means' (between four and seven) and the 'well-to-do' (eight to ten). The vast majority (73 per cent) they classed as being for the middle group, with only 1 per cent for the highest.[5] More reliable evidence has been produced from assessments based on the rateable value of given addresses in Middlesbrough hospitals, suggesting the 'class and wealth' of inpatients changed little with the arrival of private patients.[6]

The emergence of private provisions might be seen as a logical development, given the elite reputation of the larger voluntary hospitals and the common view of the alternative – poor law infirmaries – as institutions of last resort.[7] Indeed, this was the view of Charles Rosenberg in identifying a 'private patient revolution' in American hospitals at the turn of the twentieth century.[8] However, as Paul Bridgen has argued, based on King's Fund evidence for London, the British voluntary hospitals ultimately failed to become the provider of hospital services for the middle classes. He suggests that, despite the efforts of the King's Fund, a 'voluntary hospital insufficiency' in middle-class provision left the middle classes with 'little to lose' from the nationalisation of the hospitals in the NHS.[9] Taking a wider view of the patterns of provision, it is clear that the relocation of middle-class patients requiring institutional care, from the nursing home to the hospital, was only partially achieved over the early twentieth century. The crude financial sense of redirecting the efforts of the hospitals towards these private patients was rejected in favour of a continued focus on treating the sick poor of the working classes.

Five key conclusions can be drawn regarding the patterns of provision across Britain. First, that middle-class provision remained marginal in the voluntary hospitals up until nationalisation, despite some gradual growth over the early twentieth century. In line with Bridgen, this runs counter to assumptions of a fundamental shift towards a consumer-insurance system.[10] Second, that such provision was more heavily focused in the general hospitals than specialist institutions. Third, that it was more often to be found in smaller hospitals than larger ones. Fourth, entirely private hospitals were very rare. Instead, private patients were usually a small minority in the institution; while separate wards, sometimes in separate buildings, meant they were unlikely to receive treatment alongside the working classes. Finally, provision was largely provided around a few major cities, and when considered proportionately to the local population, provision appears predominantly to be a characteristic of the southern voluntary hospital sector.

As a wealthy southern city and regional medical centre, we might well expect Bristol to be a hub of private hospital provision.[11] In fact, it was quite the opposite. The number of private beds in Bristol hospitals was significantly below the national average and they were atypically concentrated in specialist institutions. To understand this we must see Bristol in its regional context, especially alongside the neighbouring city of Bath. The specialist services of Bristol's hospitals, particularly in maternity care, contributed to a dual hub split between the two cities, jointly providing hospital services to the region's middle classes. This variation in locality, size and type of hospital both explains the aytpicality of Bristol and nuances the 'insufficiency' of private provision identified by Bridgen.[12]

The scale of private provision

Britain: the national picture

In assessing the scale of private hospital provision before the NHS, we find a problematic lack of comprehensive or reliable data, with confusion common over the term 'pay bed'. It is a somewhat misleading phrase as it was increasingly the norm through the early twentieth century for most patients to pay something. Therefore all beds might be classified as pay beds.[13] This problem seems to effect both of the main contemporary national sources we have for hospital statistics: the Hospital Year-Books (which succeeded *Burdett's Charities* in the early 1930s as a compilation of annual hospital information) and the reports of the wartime regional hospital surveys conducted by the Ministry of Health and the Nuffield Provincial Hospitals Trust. In both there were

confusions in recording the number of private beds for various institutions, sometimes listing all beds as pay beds. In Bristol, for example, this
was seen in the cases of the Bristol Maternity Hospital, the Walker
Dunbar Hospital for Women and Children, and the maternity Grove
House Home.[14]

To avoid such confusions, we might turn to metropolitan bodies
such as the King's Fund; although information from an organisation
with its own policy agenda will always need to be seen in that light. The
earliest available figures on the scale of private provision in the voluntary hospital sector come from a King's Fund comparison of the number
of pay beds in 100 London hospitals in 1913 and 1933, provided confi-
dentially for parliamentarians promoting simplifying the process for
allowing private patients in hospitals where there were problems with
the wording of their charitable trust deeds. For 1913 they record 393
pay beds and 3,225 ordinary beds (a little over 10 per cent of the total).
For 1933 it was 1,389 to 4,050 (slightly over 25 per cent).[15] There can
be little doubt, however, that those 100 hospitals were highly unrepre-
sentative and presumably chosen in order to present a distorted picture
in which private provision for the middle classes was both a significant
and rapidly growing part of hospital work in the capital. If over a quarter
of beds had been private across London's 159 voluntary hospitals this
would have totalled over 4,000; rather more than the 1,573 listed in the
1933 Hospitals Year-Book. This fuller source gives the proportion of
voluntary hospital beds for private patients in the capital a little below
9 per cent.[16] Given that the King's Fund briefing papers claimed the rate
was higher than this in 1913, before twenty years of expansion, the
choice of which 100 hospitals to record – unnamed and with no criteria
given for their selection – appears little more than an exclusion of those
institutions not sharing their enthusiasm for the admission of private
patients. The King's Fund itself can hardly have been under the impression that the capital's hospitals all fitted this pattern, when they had
found from a questionnaire in 1927 that forty-one were making no
private provision whatsoever.

Despite all these gaps and uncertainties with various information
sources, some general trends are identifiable. From 1933 the Hospitals
Year-Books show a trend of growth. In absolute terms, as can be
seen from figure 4.1, the number of private beds in voluntary hospitals
across Britain increased by four-fifths in the fifteen years before the

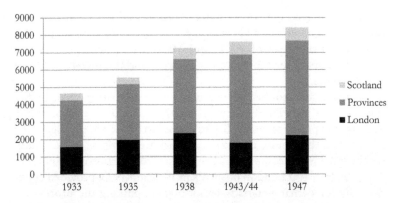

Figure 4.1 Number of private beds in Britain, 1933–47

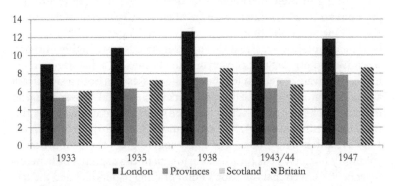

Figure 4.2 Private beds as a percentage of all voluntary hospital beds in Britain, 1933–47

introduction of the NHS. The rate of this growth, however, was much greater in the 1930s than the 1940s. Between 1933 and 1938 it increased by two-thirds, while by less than one-tenth between 1938 and 1947. A modest growth was returned after a temporary wartime slowdown, when private wards were among those reallocated under the Emergency Medical Service. This growth in private beds was slightly ahead of the growth in voluntary hospital beds in general, as shown in figure 4.2. Here there was also a clear trend of growth between 1933 and 1938, from 6 per cent in the early 1930s to around 8.5 per cent. Despite a small increase in the overall number of private beds during the war, they declined as a focus of the hospitals' work, falling back to almost early 1930s levels. Across the country the balance was restored thereafter, so the situation in the provinces on the eve of war was very similar to that on the eve of the NHS. This was not the case for the heavily bombed and evacuated capital. Although private provision was still most prominent in London's voluntary hospitals, late 1930s levels were not restored after the war either as a proportion of beds or in absolute terms.

What is harder to put a figure on is the number of private beds for middle-class patients in public hospitals. As previously discussed, the assumption that all voluntary hospital beds were private has been unhelpful. The assumption that the larger and more numerous public hospitals made no private provision has been even more unhelpful. Most directories and surveys appear to have thought this figure not worth recording, although the wartime survey of the North West region is a rare exception (discussed further below). If we treat the North West of England's private 0.27 per cent of public hospital beds as representative, we can come to a very rough projected estimate for the whole of Britain; somewhere under 4,000 private beds out of the 144,000 total in all British public hospitals. Taking this combined with the voluntary hospital figures, we can estimate that only around 3 or 4 per cent of all hospital beds before the NHS were those for the middle-class fifth of the population. While this figure should be taken only as a rough estimate, it does demonstrate clearly that provision for the middle classes was very much a fringe aspect of the pre-NHS hospitals' work.

The scale of private provision in Bristol

Bristol did not fit this pattern. Only slightly more than 2 per cent of voluntary hospital beds in the city were private in 1933.[17] In fact, the first private beds were not established in Bristol until 1926. Four years earlier, the Bristol Royal Infirmary's House Committee had prevented the introduction of private wards by accepting the opening of a new maternity ward only on the understanding that it would be exclusively for 'such patients as can pay no more than the full cost of their maintenance'.[18] Of those first private wards in Bristol, there were three double wards (two-bed rooms) charged at £5 5s 0d per week, which the King's Fund would have categorised as aimed at patients of 'moderate means'. Meanwhile, there were a further thirteen single wards (one-bed rooms) with charges of £8 8s 0d per week, which even a decade later and in

London would be classed as a level of payment appropriate for the 'well-to-do' patient.[19] This was significantly higher than the rates suggested by the Honorary Medical Staffs, which at different times was a flat rate of five guineas per week, three-to-four guineas per week, and £3 3s 0d for double wards and £4 4s 0d for single wards.[20] The implication of the higher rates put into practice is that, although limited, this earliest private hospital provision in Bristol was amongst the elite.

From this limited but elite provision in the late 1920s, the 1930s saw an increase in the number of private beds in Bristol. Although provision at the Bristol Royal Infirmary was reduced in the early 1930s from the initial nineteen beds to fifteen, other hospitals introduced private wards, as can be seen from figure 4.3. These included four (rising to six) beds at the Bristol Royal Hospital for Sick Women and Children, with charges of £3 13s 6d. The Cossham Memorial Hospital had three (reduced to two) and the Bristol Maternity Hospital for a short time had four, all charged at £4 4s 0d. The six private beds at the Bristol Homeopathic Hospital were charged at £7 7s 0d per week. The Bristol General Hospital introduced three private beds at the same time as

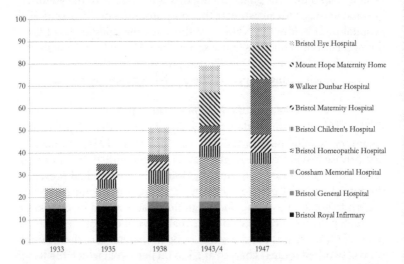

Figure 4.3 Growth in number of private beds in Bristol voluntary hospitals, 1933–47
Note: General hospitals in solid, specialist hospitals patterned.

amalgamating with the Bristol Royal Infirmary, producing a combined eighteen beds, while the Bristol Eye Hospital opened a further twelve in the late 1930s. At the close of the decade, in 1939, a new private ward of fifteen beds was opened at the Mount Hope Maternity Home, as the hospital's coverage was extended to married mothers. These figures reveal a near doubling of private hospital provision in Bristol over the second half of the 1930s.[21]

A similar system to that of the voluntary hospitals was in operation at Bristol's pre-NHS public hospitals – in particular, Southmead Hospital. A Ministry of Health survey of the city's health services in the early 1930s commented on its ten 'single wards' for 'paying patients' at a charge of £3 3s 0d per week.[22] There is little evidence of how private provision developed from this point, although we know one former patient was written to in 1941 by the city's Medical Officer of Health informing her 'that the Assessment Sub-Committee, with their authority passed a Resolution requiring you to contribute the sum of £17 2s 0d in respect of Maintenance of Self' for a period of thirty-eight days as an inpatient.[23] This shows a municipal hospital operating a private system based on a distinction between a set charge for maintenance and a separately negotiated medical fee, just as in the voluntary hospitals.[24] A notable difference in payment between the two, however, was the rate of payment. This was significantly lower at Southmead, suggesting the city's municipal general hospital was not catering for its wealthiest citizens.[25] Another difference is who requested payment. As private wards were introduced in the voluntary hospitals it became an important point for the medical staffs that they should not directly be involved in collecting funds.[26] It would appear that the city's long-serving Medical Officer of Health, Dr R.H. Parry, either had no such qualms or was convinced to set them aside. Although this might not have been standard procedure, it does suggest the provision of private hospital services was firmly embedded in the city's municipal health culture.

We might assume, given the fact that Southmead had been taken over in 1930 by the Corporation, that the introduction of this system was part of the new municipal arrangement. However, a conference organised shortly before by the Medical Officer of Health, which brought together representatives of the city's hospitals heard that, although Southmead 'was designed for the pauper sick', the poor law guardians had 'found it necessary to throw open their doors to patients of all classes'.[27] Of Southmead's 3,000 patients in 1929, 'roughly one half were not pauper patients' they heard, suggesting the patient base was increasingly similar to that of the voluntary hospitals even before municipalisation. Moreover, they were told that this change would 'remove the stigma of pauperism' from the hospital.[28] The Council's policy for admission at Southmead was explained in remarkably familiar terms: 'the sick poor would have first claim upon the accommodation at Southmead, but any citizen would have the right to apply for a bed at the Hospital, subject to the condition of paying all or part of the cost, if able.' The 1929 Local Government Act reinforced this system, making it 'the duty of the Corporation under the Act to recover the cost of treatment from all patients who are able to pay'.[29]

The fact that these patients were accommodated in the ten 'single wards' is hard to square with their aim 'to ensure that those persons who will receive from the Council by reason of their poor circumstances assistance in the form of hospital treatment shall do so in the same hospitals and under the same conditions as the rest of the citizens'.[30] At Southmead the Corporation, as the Board of Guardians before them, were aiming to provide a general hospital service with essentially the same payment system as the voluntary hospitals.

Locating private provision

Beyond the voluntary-municipal mix, there are three dimensions to the pattern of provision we should consider. The first of these is the institutional location of private beds according to the size of the hospital, which sheds light on how segregated or integrated private patients were as well as on how much private provision characterised and directed the work of the voluntary hospitals. Understanding the type of hospital (i.e. general or specialist) can help us gain some understanding of what kinds of medical treatment were being provided to middle-class patients. The third is the geographical spread of provision, revealing the extent to which middle-class treatment in the voluntary hospitals was a reality across the country.

Size of hospital

The key question here is whether provision for the middle classes was primarily located in those larger institutions, the mainstay of medical treatment for the acute sick in the area, or in those smaller ones focused on serving a certain group or service, or indeed whether provision might be spread across the two. Figure 4.4 shows the prominence of private wards in small hospitals (with fewer than 100 beds), medium-sized hospitals (with 100–199 beds), and large hospitals. Consistently we see private beds accounting for by far the largest proportion of all beds in small hospitals, and the smallest proportions in large hospitals. Although Bristol had very few private beds in medium-sized hospitals, it was in line with the national picture in having a majority in small hospitals. A rather different situation was evident in Glasgow, with two-thirds of its private beds found in large voluntary hospitals, and a further 10 per cent in a 185-bed institution.[31] However, the largest with private beds in the rest of Scotland was the Queen Mary Nursing Home, a hospital of fifty-five beds in Edinburgh. We might assume those large proportions of beds for private patients in small hospitals added up to little, with the smaller proportions in the biggest hospitals being the most significant to look at. In fact, as figure 4.5 shows, the opposite is true. In the early 1930s there were more private beds in small hospitals than in medium and large ones combined. Even as the proportion of private beds found in large hospitals increased, and that in medium and

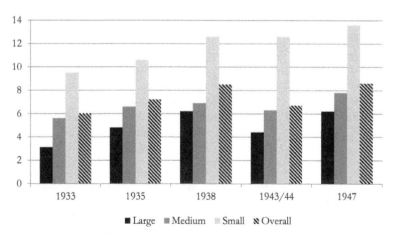

Figure 4.4 Private beds as a percentage of total provision in voluntary hospitals of different size in Britain, 1933–47

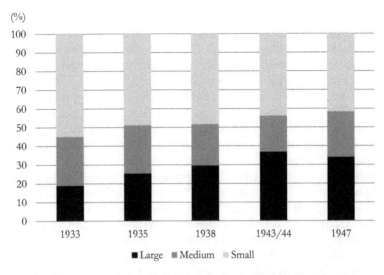

Figure 4.5 Proportion of all private beds in different size voluntary
hospitals in Britain, 1933–47

small ones decreased, over the next decade there were still more private
beds in small than large hospitals.

While the faster expansion of private wards in large hospitals in the
1940s did narrow the gap to less than 4 per cent, it is clear that middle-
class patients were readily opting for treatment in smaller institutions.
Evidently they did not share the view of Lord Moran, President of the
Royal College of Physicians, who described hospitals with fewer than
100 beds as 'much too small to fulfil the functions of a first-class hospital'.[32] Health Minister Aneurin Bevan expressed a similar opinion during
the passage of the National Health Service Bill in 1946:

> There is a tendency in some quarters to defend the very small hospital
> on the ground of its localism and intimacy, and for other rather impon-
> derable reasons of that sort, but everybody knows today that if a hospital
> is to be efficient it must provide a number of specialised services.
> Although I am not myself a devotee of bigness for bigness sake, I would
> rather be kept alive in the efficient if cold altruism of a large hospital than
> expire in a gush of warm sympathy in a small one.[33]

The larger share of private beds found in small hospitals might be explained by a great number of entirely private hospitals specialising in treating middle-class patients, if it were not for the fact that such institutions were exceedingly rare. There were of course a huge number of private nursing homes providing care for the sick; but only nine such institutions with resident medical officers existed in 1933.[34] By 1938 their number had doubled, though remained very limited at only eighteen in all of England (see table 4.1). In Scotland there were a further four. These were a hospital for women in Glasgow of sixty-seven beds and another of forty in Edinburgh, as well as an eight-bed hospital in Wick and a four-bed maternity home in Berwickshire. Eight of the eighteen in England were general hospitals, including London's Royal Masonic Hospital in Ravenscourt Park, by some way the largest with

Table 4.1 Entirely private hospitals in England, 1938

Hospital	Type	Area	Beds
Royal Masonic, Ravenscourt Park	General	London	200
Forbes Fraser Private Hospital	General	Bath	74
The Fielding Johnson	General	Leicester	43
Queen Victoria Nursing Institution	General	Wolverhampton	42
Bromhead Nursing and Maternity Home	General	Lincoln	34
St Mary's Convalescent Home	Special	Somerset	34
Leazes House Sanatorium, Wolsingham (TB)	Special	Durham	33
The John Faire, Leicester	General	Leicester	30
St Saviours for Ladies of Limited Means (Women & Children)	General	London	21
Rosehill Private Sanatorium, Penzance	Special	Cornwall	20
Ellerslie House	Special	Nottingham	18
Burton-on-Trent Nursing Institution and Maternity Home	Special	Burton-on-Trent	15
Merthyr Guest Memorial Hospital	General	Somerset	12
Duchess of Connaught Memorial, Bagshot (maternity)	Special	Surrey	7

Sources: *The Hospitals Year-Books* (London, 1933–47); Ministry of Health, Regional Hospital Services Survey Reports (London, 1945).

200 beds and no other having more than seventy-five. Combined, entirely private hospitals provided only 583 beds across England in 1938. This was a rather small 9.2 per cent of all 6,341 private beds and a measly 0.7 per cent of all 83,158 voluntary hospital beds at the time. While their number increased further to twenty-two before the introduction of the NHS, the private hospital remained in our period very much a rarity.[35]

On the basis of these figures, any notion that the voluntary hospitals were essentially private hospitals can be refuted outright. Sir Henry Charles Burdett, founder of the King's Fund, had long been amongst those calling for the introduction of a series of 'Home Hospitals'. In 1879 he laid out his proposals for 'a sort of sick lodging-house' for the middle classes, 'where they can, for a reasonable payment, secure all that their case requires, and that their means will allow'. This was to be 'the pay hospital *par excellence*.'[36] Plans in 1842 for 'a hospital for the middle classes in London' had failed 'through lack of support', and it was not until 1880 that the Home Hospital Association established such an institution in the capital. Unlike in Burdett's proposals, however, Keir Waddington has described the new institution as one where 'The pay principle was implicit and the association endeavoured to promote the contributory system.'[37] By the interwar years there was a small number of entirely private hospitals, more of the kind envisaged by Burdett. A leading example, until it was taken over by municipal authorities in the 1930s, was St Chad's Hospital for paying patients in Edgbaston, Birmingham. Its 1923 report states that they received deputations from various cities considering setting up some equivalent, including London, Glasgow, Manchester, Sheffield and Bristol.[38] Clearly they did not decide to follow suit. The Honorary Secretary of the Bristol and District Divisional Hospitals Council, John Dodd, made a similar visit twenty years later, 'in view of the urgent need for this kind of accommodation in Bristol'. However, rather than visiting an entirely private hospital, he went 'to survey the private ward accommodation' of the Bradford Royal Infirmary.[39]

The overwhelming majority of private beds were to be found in ordinary hospitals in wards of one or a very small number of beds. Far more common than an entirely private hospital, was devoting a separate floor or wing of the hospital building to middle-class patients, as with the Baker Memorial Wing of St George's Hospital in London or the

100-bed Canniesburn annexe of the Glasgow Royal Infirmary.[40] These
private wards very rarely became the main business of the hospital, with
private beds at half or more of the total in only five cases in the mid-
1930s. Combined, entirely private hospitals and those with a majority
of beds for private patients reached their peak of 3.1 per cent of all
voluntary hospitals by the establishment of the NHS.[41] Hence, even
after decades of growth in private provision, heavily subsidised working-class patients were the majority in 96.9 per cent of voluntary
hospitals.

We can see this pattern in Bristol, where there were no private hospitals. Instead, middle-class patients were typically found in one- or
two-bed private wards. As can be seen from table 4.2, there were only
two hospitals in Bristol where private beds were more than 10 per cent
of the total, and none as high as 15 per cent. This means the trend discussed above, for treating predominantly working-class patients, was
strongly reflected locally. Moreover, an overwhelming majority of all
private beds in the city, thirty-five of fifty-one, were located in small
hospitals.[42] This may have made it harder to provide the respectability

Table 4.2 General and private beds in all voluntary hospitals
in Bristol, 1938

Hospital	General	Private	
Bristol Royal Infirmary	410	15	3.5%
Bristol General Hospital	266	3	1.2%
Bristol Children's Hospital	103	6	5.5%
Cossham Memorial Hospital	98	2	2.0%
Bristol Eye Hospital	72	12	14.3%
Queen Victoria Jubilee Convalescent Home	80	0	0.0%
St Monica's Home of Rest	80	0	0.0%
Bristol Homeopathic Hospital	73	6	8.6%
Bristol Maternity Hospital	32	4	11.1%
Walker Dunbar Hospital	29	3	9.4%
Total	1,243	51	3.9%

Sources: *The Hospitals Year-Book for 1938* (London, 1938) and V. Cope, W.
Gill, A. Griffiths and G. Kelly, *Hospital Survey: The Hospital Services of the
South-Western Area* (London, 1945).

afforded by physically separating the two types of ward, ensuring middle-class and working-class patients had no need to brush up against each other.

Type of hospital

This concentration of Bristol's private beds in smaller hospitals is more understandable when bearing in mind that, bucking the national trend (see table 4.3), over two-thirds were in specialist institutions.[43] Although in the late nineteenth century private payment was far more common in specialist institutions, by 1938, after an expansion of private provision, four-fifths of private beds were to be found in general hospitals.[44] Yet in Bristol's three voluntary general hospitals combined there were only twenty private beds out of a 794-bed total (2.5 per cent).[45] This contrasts with the 100-bed private wards found at both the Manchester Royal Infirmary (13.5 per cent of the 740 beds) and the Glasgow Royal Infirmary (12.6 per cent of 794).[46] As table 4.2 shows, nearly one-quarter of the private beds in the city's voluntary hospitals were those at the Bristol Eye Hospital, where twelve beds was 14.3 per cent of the institutional total. What continued to grow in the 1940s was maternity provision, including the fifteen-bed private ward opened at the Salvation Army's Mount Hope Maternity Home in 1939 and an expansion to twenty-five private beds at the Walker Dunbar Hospital (see figure 4.4). Meanwhile, the Homeopathic Hospital was able to boast of doubling the number of births in its private wards from eight in 1936 to sixteen the following year.[47] Similarly, the private wards at the city's general hospitals may well have been used for the confinement of expectant mothers. It is clear that maternity was the driving force behind the limited private provision made by Bristol's voluntary hospitals.

This was a notable change in the decades that followed the city's first private provision at the Bristol Royal Infirmary in 1926, when mental and maternity cases were the two categories excluded.[48] However, this was a time of change for the status of hospital births in general, as they grew from under a quarter of all births in the 1920s to a majority in the 1940s.[49] Throughout the interwar years, however, it was the starting point for debate that hospital services 'should be available only for those mothers whom it was felt unwise to deliver at home, whether for medical or social reasons, and for teaching purposes.'[50] Yet some areas

Table 4.3 Private beds in local, regional and national voluntary hospitals by type and size of hospital in 1938

	Bristol		South West		England	
	General	Private	General	Private	General	Private
General	774	20 2.5%	4,716	514 9.8%	51,208	4,918 8.8%
Special	469	31 6.2%	1,550	95 5.8%	24,768	1,192 4.6%
200+	676	18 2.6%	1,596	64 3.9%	29,092	2,227 7.1%
100–199	201	8 3.8%	1,429	43 2.9%	22,431	1,440 6.0%
–99	366	35 6.4%	3,241	502 13.4%	24,453	2,443 9.1%
Total	1,243	51 3.9%	6,266	609 8.9%	75,976	6,110 7.4%

Sources: *The Hospitals Year-Book for 1938* (London, 1938); V. Cope, W. Gill, A. Griffiths and G. Kelly, *Hospital Survey: The Hospital Services of the South-Western Area* (London, 1945).

saw institutional birth become the new norm, such as Leeds where hospitals accounted for the majority of births by 1938, and for nearly two-thirds by 1946.[51] That private provision catered more extensively for these increasingly common hospital births than for other types of patients might be simply a result of greater demand, which was certainly increasing at this time. The explanation for this increased demand in the historical and sociological literature has gradually shifted towards seeing this as women's choice rather than the result of coercion on the part of medical men.[52] One factor that may well have made it possible to take up a preference for a hospital birth was the maternity benefit provisions of the National Insurance scheme. Subject to complex institutional arrangements, this covered up to thirty shillings for the confinement but nothing towards any fees for medical treatment.[53] As few women were covered by National Insurance or contributory scheme members in their own right, exemption from finding the money was afforded by virtue of her husband's employment. Moreover, while the numbers covered by National Insurance increased between the wars, so too did the rates of payment expected, which were often notably higher than the rate of the benefit. Meanwhile, the place of women within the contributory scheme movement is striking by its absence, with ordinary maternity cases usually excluded from coverage. The deeply flawed rationale given in Oxford for exclusion was that 'only a comparatively small number of people could qualify to receive the benefit, so that the spread of the cost over the whole body of contributors would be inequitable'.[54] Furthermore, the usual income-assessed barriers to ordinary wards were accompanied for maternity patients by moral ones, with separate wards typically in the maternity hospitals for married and unmarried mothers. Overall the case of maternity suggests the balance between medical, financial and social duties was different for female patients. The social was not restricted to class, but encompassed a far more varied and complex set of moral dimensions.[55]

Unfortunately we have no more detailed figures on the gender mix of private patients in Bristol hospitals. However, we do know that at Addenbrooke's Hospital in Cambridge, where the proportion of private beds was a little above the national average at 8.5 per cent in the mid-1930s, 55.3 per cent of private patients were women, 36.5 per cent were men and 8.2 per cent were children.[56] It does therefore appear that private provision was geared largely towards women, driven by though not limited to maternity care. While this maternity provision was not limited to specialist hospitals, it did much to ensure that Bristol bucked the wider general-specialist trend. The concentration of private beds in general hospitals was not only seen at the national level but also across Bristol's South West region, where around three-quarters of private beds were in general hospitals. This was not simply a consequence of general hospitals being larger, as private beds accounted for a greater share of all beds in general hospitals than in specialist ones. In Bristol, however, private beds were concentrated in and accounted for the greatest proportion of the total in small specialist hospitals (see table 4.3). This unusual situation can only be understood by considering Bristol's position as a hub of hospital provision within its region; and it is to regionalism and its complexities that we now turn.

Regional patterns

The minimal private hospital provision in Bristol complicates Daniel Fox's account of 'hierarchical regionalism', which has proved surprisingly resilient despite fierce criticism from Charles Webster on the grounds that it was a more accurate description of interwar policy than practice.[57] In most respects the city was a classic example of the regional centre for research, medical education and specialist services, around which the region's healthcare was said to be organised. This position as a clinical centre for the South West was long-established by the time it was recognised in the new regional structure of the NHS, with the Bristol Regional Hospital Board covering the entire region; not only including nearby Gloucestershire, Somerset and Wiltshire, but also reaching south to Dorset, Devon and Cornwall. Private hospital services, however, are notable by their absence. There is a clear contrast between the local and national pictures, but only by comparing the city to other regional centres and by examining the patterns of regional provision across the country can we be sure whether it was Bristol or private provision which bucked the trend. In adopting this regional view, the available data leads us to focus on voluntary hospitals and on the situation in England.

London served as a regional and national hub for medical services of all kinds, and those for private patients were far from an exception. As seen in figure 4.1, the capital was home to around one-third of all private beds in Britain and roughly one-quarter in the 1940s, when expansion in the provinces was accompanied by the significant disruptions of war. The regional surveys recorded London's South East region having four times more private beds than its nearest rival in 1938, with 3,268 to the 760 in Manchester and Liverpool's North West region.[58] The fact these two regions had the most private beds was in part a result of them being the most populous (see table 4.4). Indeed, there is a difficulty, for example, in comparing what was termed the 'London Area' (here renamed the 'South East'), which covered many populous areas near the south coast, with the largely rural 'Eastern Area' immediately to its north, which had a population more than eleven times smaller.[59] It is more useful, therefore, to look at the number of beds in relation to the region's population.

This makes a radical difference to the North West, where concentrated private provision was matched by a concentrated population. In fact, the region had a lower than average 0.117 private beds per 1,000, despite having the second largest number in absolute terms. The reverse is true for Bristol's less populous South West region, where 609 private beds were roughly twice as many per head at 0.230 per 1,000. This was almost identical to the South East's 0.231, both of which were significantly greater than the nearby Oxford region's 0.189. These three southern regions stand out as having the greatest private provision proportionate to population, while the lowest were to be found in Sheffield's East Midlands region, the Yorkshire region which included Leeds, and the North East, each with less than one bed per ten thousand. This division between north (including the Midlands and East Anglia) and south appears clear and striking. The overall English rate of private provision was 0.157 private beds per thousand population, and while the three southern regions were above this, the rest were below it.

Scotland both replicates this north–south divide and fits within it. The voluntary hospitals in the South-Eastern region of Scotland, centred on Edinburgh, had a higher proportion of private beds than those in the South-Eastern region of England, centred on London (10.5 per cent to 9.4).[60] Despite a few large private wards in Glasgow hospitals, the rate was far lower across the rest of Scotland: 6.1 per cent in the Western Region, 4.4 in the Northern Region and zero in the North-Eastern Region, although a sixty-bed private ward was under consideration for the Aberdeen Royal Infirmary. Scotland's overall 5.3 per cent

Table 4.4 Private beds in voluntary hospitals per population by English region, 1938

	Population	General beds	Private beds	Private (%)	Private beds per 1,000
South East	14,160,044	31,356	3,268	9.4	0.231
South West	2,645,980	6,266	609	8.9	0.230
Berks, Bucks & Oxon	867,140	1,753	164	8.6	0.189
Eastern Area	1,249,270	3,206	173	5.1	0.139
North West	6,480,270	11,025	760	6.4	0.117
West Midlands	4,252,920	7,411	446	5.7	0.105
North East	2,533,982	3,832	241	5.9	0.095
Yorkshire Area	2,835,065	4,773	232	4.6	0.082
East Midlands	3,965,898	6,354	217	3.3	0.055
England	*38,990,569*	*75,976*	*6,110*	*7.4*	*0.157*

Sources: *The Hospitals Year-Book for 1938* (London, 1938); John B. Hunter, R. Veitch Clark and Ernest Hart, *Hospital Survey: The Hospital Services of the West Midlands Area* (London, 1945); L.G. Parsons, S. Clayton Freyers and G.E. Godber, *Hospital Survey: The Hospital Services of the Sheffield and East Midlands Area* (London, 1945); V. Zachary Cope, W.J. Gill, Arthur Griffiths and G.C. Kelly, *Hospital Survey: The Hospital Services of the South-Western Area* (London, 1945); Ernest Rock Carling and T.S. McIntosh, *Hospital Survey: The Hospital Services of the North-Western Area* (London, 1945); William G. Savage, Claude Frankau and Basil Gibson, *Hospital Survey: The Hospital Services of the Eastern Area* (London, 1945); A.M.H. Gray and A. Topping, *Hospital Survey: The Hospital Services of London and the Surrounding Area* (London, 1945); Herbert Eason, R. Veitch Clark and W.H. Harper, *Hospital Survey: The Hospital Services of the Yorkshire Area* (London, 1945); E.C. Beevers, G.E. Gask and R.H. Parry, *Hospital Survey: The Hospital Services of Berkshire, Buckinghamshire and Oxfordshire* (London, 1945); Hugh Lett and Albert Edward Quine, *Hospital Survey: The Hospital Services of the North-Eastern Area* (London, 1945).

of voluntary hospital beds for private patients is therefore significantly lower than that for England.[61]

Beneath this broad brush stroke there were also local oddities, such as the fact that 8.9 per cent of all voluntary hospital beds in Bradford were for private patients while there were none at all in York.[62] No less odd was Bristol, a wealthy southern city and a clinical centre for its region but with very few middle-class private beds. As table 4.5 shows, Bristol had fewer private beds per head than anywhere else in the region. Instead the regional hub of middle-class hospital provision appears to have been to its south in the county of Somerset and especially in the city of Bath. Despite a population one-sixth the size of Bristol's (68,300 to 415,500 in 1938) and less than half the total number of voluntary hospital beds (680 to 1,294), Bath had more than twice as many private beds (125 to 51). This was not only a difference between two cities but also points to a clear split in this north part of the South West region, as the situation in each was echoed in their surrounding rural areas. Across the county of Somerset (including Bath) private beds accounted for 15.1 per cent of all voluntary hospital beds. Across Gloucestershire (including Bristol), it was only 5.4 per cent.

Across England private beds accounted for a smaller proportion of all beds in specialist voluntary hospitals than in general ones (4.6 per cent to 8.8 per cent), but the picture was typically different in areas serving as a regional centre. In some cases the gap was notably reduced, such as London (10.1 to 12.2). In others, such as Birmingham, it was

Table 4.5 Private beds in voluntary hospitals per population in the South West areas, 1938

	Population	General beds	Private beds	Private (%)	Private beds per 1,000
Bath	68,300	555	125	18.4	1.959
Somerset	404,600	797	116	12.7	0.287
Cornwall	308,297	443	65	12.8	0.211
Devon & Exeter	529,860	1,249	100	7.4	0.189
Wiltshire	305,900	781	55	6.6	0.180
Gloucestershire	400,120	774	64	7.6	0.160
Plymouth	211,800	424	33	7.2	0.156
Bristol	415,500	1,243	51	3.9	0.122
South West	2,644,377	6,266	609	8.9	0.230

Sources: *The Hospitals Year-Book for 1938* (London, 1938); V. Cope, W. Gill, A. Griffiths and G. Kelly, *Hospital Survey: The Hospital Services of the South-Western Area* (London, 1945).

reversed (8.3 to 7.7). In Bristol this was even more pronounced (6.2 to only 2.5). Although the former is lower than in either London or Birmingham, it was still significantly higher than the national average. Bristol was not home to a major hub in specialist hospital provision for private patients, instead it was one of a number of centres spread across the region – principally between the cities of Bristol and Bath – with notably little overlap. Beyond Bristol there were only eight private beds in hospitals for women and children in 1938, seven in Plymouth and one in Wiltshire.[63] There were fourteen private beds in ophthalmic hospitals in the region, twelve of them in Bristol and another two in Bath. The only six private beds in homeopathic hospitals were in Bristol and the only twenty private beds in an ENT hospital were in Bath.[64] As such, the regional picture of specialist hospital service provision for the middle classes is not one of a single regional centre for provision, but rather one of a cluster spread across two counties, within which Bristol played a major role.

Possible explanations

When the wartime survey sought to explain the low level of private provision in Scotland's eastern region, covering an area including Dundee to the north of Edinburgh, the report explained:

> The proportion of middle-class and wealthy population in Dundee is relatively small, and the total amount of private practice available for physicians and surgeons of consultant status correspondingly limited. Consultant practice in the rest of the region has mostly been divided between Dundee on the one hand, and Edinburgh or Glasgow on the other, the latter being easy of access.[65]

The same cannot be said of the wealthy (if unequal) city of Bristol with its large middle-class population. Three possible explanations for the extremely low level of private provision at its voluntary hospitals will therefore be considered. The first of these is simply a lack of demand for medical attention amongst the middle classes. The second is that what demand there was might have been met elsewhere – either in a non-hospital setting or at the municipal hospitals. The last is that, while the middle classes were receiving treatment in voluntary hospitals, they were prepared to travel to do so elsewhere. Given the 'dual hub' in specialist regional private provision between Bristol and Bath, it will be suggested that in this case the last of the three should be seen as the primary explanation for the startlingly low level of middle-class provision made by the city's voluntary hospitals.

Lack of demand

The simplest explanation for limited provision would be limited demand. In the case of private provision, the reason might be assumed to lie in a lower rate of illness amongst the middle-class population. This may go some way to explaining the overall rate of provision, though not obviously the divergence between the American hospitals' refocusing on private provision and the continued focus in British hospitals on the treatment of the working classes. Neither would it explain why Bristol should be a city with a large middle-class population, but with far fewer hospital beds for their treatment than seen elsewhere around the country and even its own region. Consequently, for any lack of demand to serve as an explanation, it would need to be in some way specific to the city itself.

We can look to the city's hospital contributory schemes for some gauge of interest in middle-class provision. In addition to their main business of offering a form of mutual aid designed to ensure an appropriate financial contribution was made on behalf of working-class patients, in some cases they branched out and established supplementary middle-class schemes. Across the hospital contributory schemes and the medical faculty of the hospitals in Bristol, we see a common assumption that there was a middle-class demand for securing access to private treatment. The founders of Bristol's two major hospital contributory schemes were acutely aware of the need for such a service. When the Bristol Medical Institutions Contributory Scheme (BMICS) was established in 1927 and then the Bristol Hospitals Fund in 1939, both immediately gave the matter consideration.[66] In 1929, a subcommittee of the Bristol Royal Infirmary's faculty was set up to consider the suggestion of a hospital insurance scheme for the middle classes, defined as those with incomes of over £300 per year. They envisaged that such a scheme would require annual payment into a central fund, entitling admission if taken ill and covering payments for both maintenance charges and fees for treatment.[67] This reversed the faculty's previous stance that the admission of this class of patient 'should be determined by the almoner on the individual merits of each case, & not on the basis of subscribing to any contributory scheme.'[68]

The following year the BMICS established their 'Section II' scheme 'to assist those who normally, owing to income limits, are not eligible for treatment in the public wards of the Voluntary Medical Institutions'. This would cover the member or a dependant if they 'should have to become a patient in a private ward of a hospital or a nursing home'.[69] In return for an annual contribution of one guinea per annum (or two for the inclusion of a dependant), the contributor would be entitled to 'grants-in-aid' of up to ten guineas per year for hospital expenses.[70] Over the early 1940s the Bristol Hospitals Fund would establish both an Intermediate Contributory Scheme and a Provident Fund, both offering access to private services for those earning different amounts over the general ward income limits. These middle-class schemes excluded certain categories of patient, such as the chronic sick and maternity cases, maintaining a focus on treating breadwinners and returning to them to work.[71]

As far as membership of the Bristol Hospitals Fund's middle-class Welfare Fund suggests, there was an interest in medical insurance for this section of the city's population. The middle-class section of the BHF's membership had grown to over 40 per cent by the introduction of the NHS, meaning a presence here twice that of the city's population at large.[72] This over-representation can be partially explained by the numerous other contributory schemes in Bristol without middle-class options. We might further be tempted to look to ideas of civic duty to explain middle-class membership alongside the schemes' fundraising efforts, as identified by Frank Prochaska in London and Nick Hayes in Nottingham.[73] However, these middle-class sections of contributory schemes in Bristol appear to be so heavily framed as insurance that such an explanation does not seem fitting. Their popularity suggests there was a demand for institutional treatment in times of sickness, of the kind covered, from the city's middle classes.

Alternative sites of treatment

Our second possible explanation is that medical attention may have been sought by the middle classes beyond the hospital setting. This may mean home treatment by general practitioners, and for those not signed up to a contributory scheme there would have been a clear financial incentive to avoid hospital treatment. While £3 would be a modest charge for a private bed in a voluntary hospital (with medical or surgical fees expected in addition), the typical charge for a doctor's home visit in the 1930s would range between one-sixth and one-twelfth of that amount.[74]

It appears the introduction of the National Insurance panel system in 1911 and its interwar expansion, when it came to cover the majority of the adult male population, did little to diminish private practice. Although Lloyd George's 'ambulance wagon' speech had vividly painted a picture of the neglected working-class need for medical attention, in 1926 the BMA estimated that general practitioners made more visits to private than panel patients.[75] We might assume demand for hospital treatment, at least in the leading voluntary hospitals, would be generated by their reputation as elite and pioneering institutions. While George Bernard Shaw had commented in 1911 that 'the rank and file of doctors are no more scientific than their tailors', by 1926 the Bristol Royal Infirmary, for example, was engaging in work of 'immense importance' treating 'supposedly incurable' cancer cases.[76] Yet, with the exception of maternity cases, middle-class patients in Bristol appear to have received treatment in the hospitals only relatively rarely. The explanation perhaps rests in the fact that the city's general practitioners were well-placed to cater for the middle classes beyond the hospital. We can see this from the geographical concentration of their premises in its wealthier suburbs to the west and north, such as Clifton, Redland and Westbury-on-Trym.[77] This was the opposite of the small town North American situation where Charles Rosenberg found 'the intractable reality of longer distances underlining the hospital's appeal', as well as supposed clinical benefits, prompting practitioners to encourage hospital treatment to their patients.[78] The location of dozens of surgeries within each of the city's wealthiest areas may have acted as a buffer against such a change in Bristol.

The proximity of private surgeries to the hospitals was no coincidence. It was very much the norm for the honorary medical staffs of the voluntary hospitals to also keep private practice.[79] For example, Dr Patrick Watson-Williams was the Bristol Royal Infirmary's first Honorary Aurist and Laryngologist, and later Honorary Consulting Surgeon in the Ear, Nose and Throat Department until his death in 1938.[80] This was a major department, which treated around one-in-ten inpatients and nearly as high a proportion of non-casualty outpatients.[81]

Throughout this busy period of hospital work he maintained a private surgery a little over a mile away from the hospital, in the middle of Clifton Village.[82] This was normal practice. All sixteen of the visiting consultants listed as medical officers in the Bristol Royal Hospital's 1939 report were also listed with private surgeries in the local directory's medical list for the same year.[83] All of these surgeries, some shared or with shared consulting rooms, were located within a small area in the centre of Clifton. Although they worked both in the hospital and with private patients, there appears to have been little appetite for bringing the two together through middle-class admissions.

Another alternative might have been for the middle-class patient to seek care in an institution other than a hospital, specifically a nursing home. Indeed, Lindsay Granshaw has noted that the development of private hospital medicine 'ran alongside the establishment in Britain of numerous nursing-homes', which she describes as 'effectively small private hospitals for the middle classes'.[84] Once again, in Bristol these tended to be found in wealthy areas, with nearly one-third of all those in the city located in Clifton.[85] Of the thirty-six nursing homes operating in and near Bristol in 1934, twenty-one advertised as offering medical services, nineteen maternity, seventeen chronic, seven surgical, two convalescent or rest, one acute and another nervous disease services.[86] Although no figures are available for their number of beds, it is likely that combined they were far greater than those for private patients in the city's hospitals.

As with general practitioners, however, nursing homes suffered from rather contrasting reputations. In 1935, a parliamentary debate on paying patients revealed an assumption held by many in the House of Lords that there must be a demand for middle-class beds in voluntary hospitals specifically because of the poor standard of the private nursing homes. Amongst them was the Labour peer Lord Sanderson, who declared 'many nursing homes' to be 'very bad and most of them very expensive', as well as not being equipped for increasingly technologically elaborate and costly procedures.[87] From the other side of the chamber, the Earl of Malmesbury spoke of a widespread and 'increasing horror – I say it with all respect – of nursing homes'.[88] By contrast, some of the elite nursing homes were commonly known as private hospitals despite having no resident medical staff, such as St Mary's and St

Brenda's in Clifton. These nursing homes branded as private hospitals would have been well-positioned to meet middle-class demand beyond the wards of the voluntary hospitals.

Certainly there were very few middle-class beds in Bristol's voluntary hospitals and likely many more in the city's great many nursing homes, but we should consider what alternative hospital admissions might have been possible. If the middle classes were, in fact, being treated in hospital when sick before the NHS, then there are two remaining possible explanations. One is that it might not have been the voluntary hospitals at all where they were receiving treatment, that is to say the middle classes may have been catered for in the municipal hospitals. Indeed, we know that both before and after appropriation, Southmead Hospital was making limited provision for private patients at a moderate rate.[89] With ten private beds in 1933, the city's public sector accounted for two-fifths of the total.[90] Moreover, we do know that such practices continued into the 1940s.[91]

The scale of this later provision in Bristol or more widely, however, remains unclear. A recent major work on interwar municipal medicine makes only passing reference to public hospitals taking fee-paying private patients.[92] Contemporary sources were less likely to record municipal private beds than those in the voluntary hospitals, with some of the regional wartime surveys not including any such figure and others giving only patchy coverage. This was most likely caused by the same confusion over the definition of a 'pay bed' as with the figures for some voluntary hospitals, suggesting payment in the ordinary wards of public hospitals was normal practice by this time. The figures that were included in these reports suggest only one region – the North West of England – fully counted private beds in municipal hospitals. They counted large wards in former workhouses (Crumpsall's thirty beds and Withington's forty-six beds in Manchester, and Birch Hill's twenty-six beds in Rochdale) as well as two municipal maternity hospitals with six beds (the Municipal Maternity Home in Warrington) and eight beds (Helm Case Maternity Home in Kendal).[93] As in the voluntary hospitals, the North West figures show private provision in the municipal hospitals located typically in general hospitals and, when in specialist institutions, those were most commonly maternity hospitals.

In total this comes to 116 private beds in the North West municipal hospitals, a notable amount but still only 13 per cent of private beds in the region's voluntary and public hospitals combined. Yet we cannot be sure if Bristol (or any other part of the country) saw the same proportion of private beds located in public hospitals, since no 'pay beds' were recorded for any of Bristol's public hospitals (and only a scattered few in other regions) despite the fact we know Southmead took private patients. However, if the number of private beds at Southmead remained unchanged over the 1930s, then the public–voluntary split would be very similar in Bristol to that recorded in the North West. Whereas some modest growth may have gone unrecorded and uncommented upon, it is highly unlikely that Bristol's public hospitals saw an expansion of private provision on a scale adequate to explain the local shortage of private beds in the voluntary hospitals.

Travelling for treatment

Of the three possible explanations considered, only alternative admission to private nursing homes appears convincing. Yet there is no evidence that this was a bigger factor in Bristol than in other cities. We must therefore turn to our final possible explanation, which is the complex position of Bristol within the region, to can gain some understanding of this unusual situation. This suggests the middle classes of Bristol were prepared to travel to receive treatment in voluntary hospitals elsewhere.

If we look first at patients from all wards, both general and private, we find that the majority of patients at the Bristol Royal Infirmary in 1930, for example, were local to the institution: 6,173 of the year's 8,734 patients were listed as being from Bristol and District. Most of the remainder were from either Gloucestershire or Somerset, including large numbers from both the nearby areas of Avonmouth and Sea Mills (103) and Shirehampton (124). There were only occasionally patients from as far afield as Worcester, Swindon and Salisbury, and a much larger number (293) from Wales.[94] Overall, patients were prepared to travel to Bristol when necessary.

For middle-class patients the necessity would have been to travel the distance of a little over ten miles, between Bristol and Bath, in both directions. While Bath might appear the regional centre for middle-class medicine from the far greater number of private beds in its hospitals, we should not overlook which hospitals had private wards. From Bristol, the nearest private bed in a specialist ENT hospital was in Bath.

From Bath, the closest private bed in a homeopathic or maternity hospital was to be found in Bristol.[95] Bristol was not displaced by Bath, therefore, but was in fact the junior partner in a dual hub of private hospital provision in the South West region; and this should be seen as the primary reason for the startlingly low level of middle-class provision made in the city's voluntary hospitals.

This becomes clearer still when we combine the figures (shown in table 4.5) for the counties of Gloucestershire and Somerset, including the cities of Bristol and Bath respectively, revealing 356 of this wider area's 3,369 voluntary hospital beds were private. At 10.6 per cent this proportion of beds for private patients is higher than average and not so far behind the 12.6 per cent found in London.[96] With 0.276 private beds per 1,000 people in the two counties, the middle-class population was better catered for than in most parts of the country. Middle-class patients were simply not treated alongside working-class patients. We already know they were treated in separate wards, commonly on other floors or in another building, but in this case also often away from the city. Where Bristol was very much the regional centre for the hospital treatment of the working classes, the middle classes typically went elsewhere.

Pay beds after 1948

Placing our focus on the idea and the act of payment both heightens and diminishes the significance of 1948 as a watershed in the history of British healthcare. Despite the principle of medical services free at the point of use, patient payment has always had some role within the NHS.[97] Indeed, those limited 'pay beds' present in the pre-NHS hospitals as the only means of securing treatment for middle-class patients were continued and became a means for those with cash to opt out of the public health service. Although private practice was entrenched and even encouraged within the NHS, it remained contentious, leading to private surgery fees being capped in 1953 at seventy-five guineas, although allowed to rise to 125 guineas in exceptional circumstances.[98] As the Teaching Hospital Association commented in the mid-1970s: 'Private practice, when conducted in hospitals, has always been a matter for controversy ever since the voluntary hospitals first began to provide beds for paying patients and so, if it continues, it will certainly and unavoidably remain so.'[99]

It was at this time that Harold Wilson and his Secretary of State for Social Services, Barbara Castle, launched the only serious attempt to abolish them. She instructed the new Health Services Board to phase them out, starting with those under-utilised, but with only modest success. When Labour took office in 1974 there were almost 5,000 pay beds in the NHS.[100] When Margaret Thatcher arrived in Downing Street five years later there remained 3,000 pay beds in NHS hospitals across England and Wales. Less than two months after taking office it was declared:

> The Government believes that people who wish to do so should be free to make arrangements for their private medical treatment and intends to repeal the legislation for the phasing-out of pay beds which was introduced by the previous Government. The Health Services Board will be abolished and the Social Services Secretary's power to allow NHS hospitals to be used for private practice will be restored.[101]

Despite a 'ceiling' on the amount of private practice and a promise of legislation to ensure, echoing the calls of the 1930s, 'that services for private patients should not prejudice services for NHS patients', the place of pay beds within NHS hospitals was reasserted. Yet, just as numbers had been low in Bristol before 1948, so they continued to be thereafter. By the mid-1970s there were just six under-used pay beds at the new Bristol Maternity Hospital and another three at Southmead Hospital.[102] A few years later, after thirty years of the NHS, there were none left in the city.

Conclusion

In some respects Bristol bucked regional and national trends in its hospital provision for middle-class patients, perhaps surprisingly given its large middle-class population and clear status as a regional centre for hospital services. Yet, before the NHS, the city's general voluntary hospitals never had more than twenty private beds between them, even though such hospitals were where the overwhelming majority of private beds were to be found nationally. At the same time it was home to a higher than average share of private beds in specialist institutions, in common with other regional hospital centres, such as Birmingham.

Understanding these contradictions and idiosyncrasies requires us to place the local situation not only within the national context, but also to consider the city within the regional picture.

Ultimately, however, the evidence presented in this chapter points to a relatively straightforward conclusion: treating the middle classes was a marginal aspect of the services provided by the pre-NHS hospitals, with access limited to the 3 or 4 per cent of hospital beds set aside for them. Middle-class patients were treated in voluntary hospitals more often than public ones, but even there private beds were never as much as 9 per cent of the total. While these private beds took over more of the hospital than usual in London, in Bristol it was the opposite. Placing Bristol in its regional context brings the level of private provision into line with a general southern concentration. The fact this happened away from the region's hospital centre highlights the degree to which the city's hospitals remained un-democratised in this period. The limited provision made for the middle classes, especially striking in Bristol, supports Paul Bridgen's argument that the voluntary hospitals ultimately failed to become the provider of hospital services to the middle classes.[103] However, this is not to say they were conservative institutions, reluctant to adapt to a new era. The small but steady stream of middle-class patients admitted was in itself a notable change and part of a wider reinterpretation of the patient contract. What remained consistent, however, was what group of society primarily constituted 'the hospital class of patient.'[104]

This traditionalism only characterised one part of a dual system that allowed the medical profession to combine hospital work and private practice. It was an arrangement to which the honorary consultants and private patients alike appear to have been wedded. Whether there was less demand amongst the middle classes than might have been assumed, they were being treated elsewhere or a combination of the two, what is clear is that the treatment of private patients was far from a central function of either the public or the voluntary hospitals before the NHS.

Notes

1 Henry Burdett, *Pay Hospitals and Paying Wards throughout the World: Facts in Support of a Re-Arrangement of the English System of Medical Relief* (London: J.&A. Churchill, 1879), p. 85.

2 BSC, DM980 (30), Bristol Hospitals Commission 1941, Evidence of the Bristol Hospitals Fund, appendix 1; and DM980 (12), Income Limits file, Extracts from General and Purposes Committee minutes on Income Limits, 27 August 1943.

3 John Stevenson, *British Society 1914–1945* (Harmondsworth: Penguin, 1984), p. 119.

4 London Metropolitan Archives [hereafter LMA], A/KE/185, King's Fund, Voluntary Hospitals (Paying Patients) Bill [hereafter VHPPB], Draft Statement for the Information of the Promoters (confidential), revised draft, 27 March 1935.

5 LMA, A/KE/185, King's Fund, VHPPB, Information for Promoters (confidential), 27 March 1935.

6 Richard Lewis, Robina Nixon, and Barry M. Doyle, *Health Services in Middlesbrough: North Ormesby Hospital 1900–1948* (Middlesbrough: Centre for Local Historical Research, University of Teesside, 1999), pp. 43–5.

7 For a discussion of how these factors led to the diversification of hospital funding, see Martin Gorsky, John Mohan, and Martin Powell, 'The Financial Health of Voluntary Hospitals in Interwar Britain', *Economic History Review*, 55:3 (2002), 533–57.

8 Charles Rosenberg, *The Care of Strangers: The Rise of America's Hospital System* (New York: Johns Hopkins University Press, 1987), pp. 237–61.

9 Paul Bridgen, 'Voluntary Failure, the Middle Classes, and the Nationalisation of the British Voluntary Hospitals, 1900–1946' in Bernard Harris and Paul Bridgen (eds), *Charity and Mutual Aid in Europe and North America since 1800* (London: Routledge, 2007), pp. 216 and 228. Given its focus on the King's Fund, this sits well alongside F.K. Prochaska, *Philanthropy and the Hospitals of London: The King's Fund, 1897–1990* (Oxford: Clarendon Press, 1992). Lewis, *et al.*, *Health Services* offers some local analysis, although the existing literature provides little context for such an investigation.

10 See Steven Cherry, 'Beyond National Health Insurance. The Voluntary Hospitals and Hospital Contributory Schemes: A Regional Study', *Social History of Medicine*, 5:3 (1992), 455–82.

11 V. Zachary Cope *et al.*, 'Hospital Survey: The Hospital Services of the South-Western Area' (London: HMSO, 1945), p. 128.

12 Bridgen, 'Voluntary Failure', p. 216.

13 It is for this reason that the term 'private bed' is used here instead of 'pay beds'.

14 For more details of these confusions see George Campbell Gosling, 'Charity and Change in the Mixed Economy of Healthcare in Bristol,

1918–1948', unpublished PhD thesis, Oxford Brookes University, 2011, pp. 249–52.

15 King's Fund, VHPPB, Information for Promoters.

16 *The Hospitals Year-Book* (1933).

17 *Ibid.*

18 BRI, Faculty Minutes, 17 February 1926.

19 BRI, 29 June 1926.

20 BRI, 16 February 1928, 17 February 1926 and 19 October 1932.

21 For Mount Hope figures, see Cope *et al.*, 'Hospital Survey', p. 32. For other private beds figures, see *The Hospitals Year-Books*, 1933–47.

22 TNA, MH 66/1068, 'County Borough of Bristol' by Allan C. Parsons (Ministry of Health, 1932), p. 142.

23 BRO, 35717/I/7/d, Notice to Miss L Morse at the Almshouse from Public Health Committee asking for contribution to cost of stay at Southmead Hospital 1941.

24 George Campbell Gosling, '"Open the Other Eye": Payment, Civic Duty and Hospital Contributory Schemes in Bristol, c.1927–1948', *Medical History*, 54:4 (2010), 477. See also Lewis *et al.*, p. 7; and Cherry, 'Insurance', p. 470.

25 King's Fund 'Information for the Promoters'.

26 George Campbell Gosling, 'The Patient Contract in Bristol's Voluntary Hospitals, c.1918–1929', *University of Sussex Journal of Contemporary History*, 11 (2007), 8.

27 BRO, BCM, 1 January, 1930, p. 253.

28 *Ibid.*, p. 250.

29 *Ibid.*, p. 251. Further evidence for continuity is offered by the Ministry of Health's report, which gave numbers for private patients before and after appropriation. See Parsons, 'Bristol', p. 142.

30 BCM, Report of the Health Committee, 1 April 1930.

31 C.F.W. Illingworth, J.M. Mackintosh and R.J. Peters, *Scottish Hospitals Survey: Report on the Western Region* (Edinburgh: Department of Health for Scotland, HMSO, 1946), p. 58.

32 Lord Moran, HL Deb 16 April 1946, vol. 140, cc. 822–823.

33 Aneurin Bevan, HC Deb, 30 April 1946, vol. 422, c. 44.

34 *Hospitals Year-Book* (London: CBHI, 1933).

35 *Hospitals Year-Books* (1933–47).

36 Burdett, *Pay Hospitals*, pp. 104 and 131. For Home Hospital proposals see ch. 11, pp. 101–30.

37 Keir Waddington, *Charity and the London Hospitals 1850–1898* (Woodbridge: Boydell Press, 2000), p. 89.

38 LMA, St Chad's Hospital for paying patients, *Report for 1923*, p. 8

39 TNA, MH77/13, John Dodd to Ernest Brown MP, 9 June 1943.
40 John Pickstone describes a similar situation at the Manchester Royal Infirmary in *Medicine and Industrial Society: A History of Hospital Development in Manchester and Its Region* (Manchester: Manchester University Press, 1985), pp. 259 and 265.
41 *Hospitals Year-Books* (1933–48).
42 *Hospitals Year-Book* (1938); Cope *et al.*, 'Hospital Survey'.
43 *Ibid.*
44 See Waddington, *Charity and the London Hospital*, pp. 91–3.
45 Cope, *et al.*, *Survey*.
46 *Hospitals Year-Book* (1938), p. 204; Pickstone, *Manchester*, p. 265; C.F.W. Illingworth, J.M. Mackintosh and R.J. Peters, *Scottish Hospitals Survey: Report on the Western Region* (Edinburgh: Department of Health for Scotland, HMSO, 1946), p. 58.
47 Bristol Homeopathic Hospital, *Report for 1937*, p. 29.
48 BRI, Faculty Minutes, 29 June 1926.
49 Tania McIntosh, *A Social History of Maternity and Childbirth: Key Themes in Maternity Care* (London: Routledge, 2012), p. 64; Jane Lewis, *The Politics of Motherhood: Child and Maternal Welfare in England, 1900–1939* (London: McGill-Queens University Press, 1980), p. 120.
50 Elizabeth Peretz, 'Maternal and Child Welfare in England and Wales between the Wars: A Comparative Regional Study', unpublished PhD thesis, Middlesex University, 1992, p. 73.
51 Barry M. Doyle, *The Politics of Hospital Provision in Early 20th-Century Britain* (London: Pickering & Chatto, 2014), pp. 101–2.
52 For the coercion view see also the work of Ann Oakley, including *Women Confined: Towards a Sociology of Childbirth* (New York: Schocken Books, 1980). For more recent works affording greater agency to women, see Lara Marks, '"They're magicians": Midwives, Doctors and Hospitals: Women's Experience of Childbirth in Eat London and Woolwich in the Interwar Years', *Oral History*, 23 (1995), 46–53; McIntosh, *Maternity and Childbirth*; Alison Nuttall, 'Taking "Advantage of the Facilities and Comforts … Offered": Women's Choice of Hospital Delivery in Interwar Edinburgh' in Janet Greenlees and Linda Bryder (eds), *Western Maternity 1880–1990* (London: Pickering & Chatto, 2013), pp. 65–80.
53 See Doyle, *Politics of Hospital Provision*, pp. 66, 133 and 192–3.
54 Radcliffe Infirmary, *Annual Report* (1924); Barnett House Survey Committee, *Social Services in Oxford: A Survey of the Social Services in the Oxford District, Volume 2* (Oxford: Oxford University Press, 1940), p. 141, cited in Peretz, 'Maternal and Child Welfare', p. 77.

55 For a further discussion of the limited choices of the pre-NHS pregnant patient-consumer see George Campbell Gosling, 'The Birth of the Pregnant Patient-Consumer? Payment, Paternalism and Maternity Hospitals in Early Twentieth-Century England' in Jennifer Evans and Ciara Meehan (eds), *Perceptions of Pregnancy from the Seventeenth to the Twentieth Century* (London: Palgrave Macmillan, 2016).

56 Addenbrooke's Hospital, *Annual Reports for 1935 and 1936*.

57 Daniel M Fox, *Health Policies, Health Politics: The British and American Experience, 1911–1965* (Princeton: Princeton University Press, 1986); Charles Webster, 'Conflict and Consensus: Explaining the British Health Service', *Twentieth Century British History*, 1:2 (1990), 115–51.

58 A.M.H. Gray and A. Topping, *Hospital Survey: The Hospital Services of London and the Surrounding Area* (London: HMSO, 1945); Ernest Rock Carling and T.S. McIntosh, *Hospital Survey: The Hospital Services of the North-Western Area* (London: HMSO, 1945).

59 Gray and Topping, *London Survey*, p. 1; Willam G. Savage, Claude Frankau and Basil Gibson, *Hospital Survey: The Hospital Services of the Eastern Area* (London: HMSO, 1945), p. 1.

60 J.W. Struthers and H.E. Seiler, *Scottish Hospitals Survey: Report on the South-Eastern Region* (Edinburgh: Department of Health for Scotland, HMSO), pp. 57–104.

61 Scottish figures gleaned from R.S. Aitken and H.H. Thomson, *Scottish Hospitals Survey: Report on the Northern Region* (Edinburgh: Department of Health for Scotland, HMSO, 1946); R.S. Aitken and H.H. Thomson, *Scottish Hospitals Survey: Report on the Eastern Region* (Edinburgh: Department of Health for Scotland, HMSO, 1946); R.S. Aitken and H.H. Thomson, *Scottish Hospitals Survey: Report on the North-Eastern Region* (Edinburgh: Department of Health for Scotland, HMSO, 1946); C.F.W. Illingworth, J.M. Mackintosh and R.J. Peters, *Scottish Hospitals Survey: Report on the Western Region* (Edinburgh: Department of Health for Scotland, HMSO, 1946).

62 Herbert Eason, R. Veitch Clark and W.H. Harper, *Hospital Survey: The Hospital Services of the Yorkshire Area* (London: HMSO, 1945).

63 Cope *et al.*, 'Hospital Survey', pp. 164, 178 and 188.

64 *Ibid.*, pp. 172 and 178.

65 R.S. Aitken and H.H. Thomson, *Scottish Hospitals Survey: Report on the Eastern Region* (Edinburgh: Department of Health for Scotland, 1946), pp. 2–3.

66 BMICS, *Report for 1929*, p. 6; *Western Daily Press* and *Bristol Mirror*, 20 July 1939.

67 BRI, Faculty Minutes, 18 September 1929.

68 *Ibid.*, 16 March 1927.
69 BMICS, *Report for 1932*, inside front cover.
70 BMICS, *Report for 1930*, p. 2.
71 BMICS, *Report for 1937*, inside back cover.
72 Bristol Reference Library, Bristol Hospitals Fund, Reports.
73 Prochaska, *King's Fund*; Nick Hayes, ' "Our Hospitals"? Voluntary Provision, Community and Civic Consciousness in Nottingham Before the NHS', *Midland History*, 37:1 (2012), 84–105.
74 An estimate of 1930s GP home visit fees ranging from 5s 0d to 10s 6d, based on the advertisement columns of the *British Medical Journal*, is presented in *ibid.*, p. 88.
75 David Lloyd George, 'The Insurance of the People', Birmingham speech, 10 June 1911 (London, 1911); Anne Digby and Nick Bosanquet, 'Doctors and Patients in an Era of National Health Insurance and Private Practice, 1913–1938', *Economic History Review*, 41:1 (1988), 74–5 and 88.
76 George Bernard Shaw, 'Preface on Doctors' to *The Doctor's Dilemma* in *Pygmalion and Three Other Plays* (New York: Barnes & Noble, 2004), p. 191; BRI, *Report for 1926*, p. 10. On the treatment see also A.T. Todd, 'A Note on the Action of a Lead-Selenium Colloid on Cancer', *Lancet*, 12 March 1927, p. 575.
77 Bristol Directory 1919, pp. 866–9; Bristol Directory 1923, pp. 949–52; Bristol Directory 1930, pp. 1030–4; Bristol Directory 1939, pp. 1320–5.
78 Rosenberg, *Care of Strangers*, p. 248.
79 See Anne Digby, *Making a Medical Living: Doctors and Patients in the English Market for Medicine, 1720–1911* (Cambridge: Cambridge University Press, 1994), p. 125.
80 BRI, *Report for 1938*, p. 15.
81 *Ibid.*, p. 36.
82 Wright's and Kelly's annual directories list Dr Watson-Williams's surgery at 2 Rodney Place, Clifton Down Road.
83 BRH, *Report for 1939*, p. 12; Bristol Directory 1939, pp. 1320–5.
84 Lindsay Granshaw, 'The Hospital' in W.F. Bynum and Roy Porter (eds), *Companion Encylopedia of the History of Medicine* (London: Routledge, 1993), vol. 2, p. 1194.
85 This is in keeping with the trends noted in Martin Powell, 'Coasts and Coalfields: The Geographical Distribution of Doctors in England and Wales in the 1930s', *Social History of Medicine*, 18:2 (2005), 245–63.
86 *Nursing Homes 1934*, pp. 83–5.
87 Lord Sanderson, HL Deb 2 April 1935, vol. 96, c. 467.
88 Earl of Malmesbury, HL Deb 2 April 1935, vol. 96, c. 476.
89 BRL, BCM, Report of the Health Committee, 26 September 1933.

90 Parsons, 'Bristol', p. 142.
91 BRO, 35717/I/7/d, Notice to Miss L Morse at the Almshouse from Public Health Committee asking for contribution to cost of stay at Southmead Hospital 1941.
92 Alysa Levene *et al.*, *From Cradle to Grave: Municipal Provision in Interwar England and Wales* (Bern: Peter Lang, 2011), p. 134.
93 Ernest Rock Carling and TS McIntosh, 'Hospital Survey: The Hospital Services of the North-Western Area' (London: HMSO, 1945), pp. 156, 160, 162, 172, 174 and 178.
94 BRI, *Report for 1930*, pp. 45–6.
95 Cope *et al.*, 'Hospital Survey', pp. 164–96.
96 *Hospitals Year-Book* (1938).
97 See John Eversley, 'The History of NHS Charges', *Contemporary British History*, 15:2 (2001), 53–75.
98 MRC, MSS.2920/847/26/5: Ministry of Health, Pay-Bed Regulations Revised: Some Reductions in Hospital Charges Likely, 18 March 1953.
99 Fourth Report of the Expenditure Committee: 'NHS Facilities for Private Patient', p. 295 cited in Department of Health and Social Security, The Separation of Private Practice from National Health Service Hospitals: A Consultative Document', September 1974, Appendix A.
100 MRC, MSS.2920/847.306.1: Department of Health and Social Security, The Separation of Private Practice from National Health Service Hospitals: A Consultative Document', September 1974; MSS.2920/847.306.3: Department of Health and Social Security, Higher Charges for Private Patients in NHS, 8 March 1978.
101 MRC, MSS.2920/847.306/4: Department of Health and Social Security, 'Private Practice of Medicine – Government Announces its Proposals', 25 June 1979.
102 MRC, SA/MWF/C.22: Box 20, Department of Health and Social Security, 'Hospitals or Groups of Hospitals in England Where in 1975 and 1976 the Occupancy of Private Pay Beds Was No Higher than 50% of the Current Number of Beds Authorised'.
103 Bridgen, 'Voluntary Failure'.
104 BCM, 10 October 1933, Report of the Health Committee, 26 September 1933.

5

The meaning of payment

The most dramatic change the NHS made to most people's everyday lives was not to provide them with medical care free at the point of use. Before 1948 hospitals had arrangements in place for this to be guaranteed to anyone for whom paying would cause financial hardship; and beyond the hospital it was not uncommon for a doctor's conscience to render him (or occasionally her) unable to charge poorer patients. Across working-class communities many who would have been expected to pay something turned to mutual aid schemes to ensure doctors' visits or hospital stays without a bill, while National Insurance made a similar arrangement compulsory for a growing number of workers in certain industries. Nor did the NHS open up greater provision. No new hospitals were built for more than a decade and the 'appointed day' did not herald the end of the dreaded waiting list. What the NHS changed was that it removed entirely questions of payment from the doctor–patient encounter. Moreover, it enshrined within commonly held notions of British citizenship that this should be so.

Just as the absence of payment after 1948 was deeply imbued with meaning, so too was the act of paying the hospital before the NHS. It was an act firmly embedded in the social relations that had always governed medical charity, even as these underwent significant changes over the early twentieth century. The previous two chapters examined the arrival in the hospital of patient payments and the almoner, contributory schemes and the middle-class patient, and how they became commonplace in the interwar years. It is typically assumed that these changes undermined or even ended philanthropy as the organising principle of the voluntary hospitals.[1] Yet, as we have already seen, practical changes that moved away from what we might expect of philanthropy were accompanied by others that safeguarded and even reinforced various core principles. While direct payments became the norm, the almoner granted notable reductions and exemptions on a means-tested basis. Although the middle classes accounted for a growing proportion of the patient base, provision for them was limited across the hospital sector, marginal within the institution and largely restricted geographically to the south of England. Even the radical break supposedly offered by mutualist contributory schemes looks rather less radical when we focus on their place within the hospital. Despite the image of insurance, membership conferred no new rights. Paying in to a contributory scheme was an opt-out of the almoner's assessment, which determined the term of access, but not access itself. Admission continued to be a medical decision regardless. However, the almoner system did more than provide a philanthropic safeguard to limit the growing commercial activities in the voluntary hospitals. It was, in fact, a reassertion of the social dynamics than underpin philanthropy itself.

The common expectation that money has a corrosive effect – that economic concerns will ultimately trump all else – was not borne out.[2] Yet payment and philanthropy did not merely find an accommodation. These new developments were incorporated into a revised understanding of medical philanthropy. In considering this, two dimensions of the hospitals' patient payment schemes will be focused upon in this chapter. The first is the social relations within which they were embedded. Some old and persistent ideas about the social function of money in the modern world tell us we should find a great levelling when payment enters a social encounter. Social distinctions should fall by the wayside in favour of those between able and unable to pay. On the contrary, instead of an anonymous and inflexible price tag attached to care, arrangements for payment were grafted on to the social classifications of patients. The distinctions in payment served to reinforce the differential (if not always deferential) class relations at the core of philanthropy. In the past these class distinctions had been enacted by providing a separate, institutional space where the sick poor would receive treatment. Admission to the hospital itself had been an act of separation. As technological advances and rising costs led the middle classes to arrive in the hospital as patients, this *class differentiation* became an internal event. The working classes submitted to a new form of charitable assessment or demonstrated thrift to secure the terms of their admission. The middle classes paid at a rate that not only covered the cost of their treatment but also served as a donation to support that of poorer patients. Payment in the doctor–patient relationship continued along traditional class lines, with working-class patients treated on an honorary basis and middle-class patients agreeing a fee. In many ways, the old social order survived.

Moreover, the payment schemes were a means to instil a moral-financial code around the use and abuse of the voluntary hospitals. A notable insight of anthropologists and sociologists has been that moral schemes are broadcast by economic activities – not only those designed to make a profit, but also spending, saving, lending, gifting, begging, accepting and refusing monies.[3] The almoner's mediation of the complex boundaries between payment and philanthropy did exactly this. The new system was not only embedded in social relations but also in social attitudes and values, including the different expectations of working- and middle-class patients. This is rather different from the democratic ideal of the NHS – comprehensive and universal – where working- and middle-class patients are treated together and on the same terms. Middle-class patients may have entered the hospitals during the interwar years, while local reforms provided something akin to a comprehensive service in some areas, including Bristol.[4] However, working- and middle-class patients were neither treated alongside each other nor on the same terms. The physical and ideological division of patients on grounds of class (assumed to be unproblematically equivalent to levels of household income) held out against a gradual move towards universalism.

The principle, termed here *economic reciprocalism*, is the second dimension. The moral code of Victorian philanthropy was one of moral reform, while the scientific charity movement sought to focus efforts on changing recipients' behaviours while stamping out indiscriminate giving.[5] The early days of the almoner profession seem to be characterised by this same mission, weeding out the 'abuse' of the middle classes seeking free treatment at the expense of the hospital, encouraging provident saving amongst those who were otherwise socially and morally deserving of free or subsidised care. However, this made way for a reformulation of medical philanthropy more in keeping with the coming collectivist age. Just as charitable provision was differentiated rather than exclusively for the poor, the expectation became that paying in was the civic duty of all but the poorest. As hospital provision became a mass operation, less deeply rooted in the communities being served, there was less hope of reforming social conduct in familiar ways.[6] Payment, however, offered a new opening into household management. Making a financial contribution was a shortcut to wider habits of saving and spending, while the almoner's assessment opened up the family's habits to the scrutiny of a philanthropic professional. Paying in, or more importantly being prepared to, became the new staple for demonstrating deservingness in medical charity.

In order to reform philanthropy in this manner, however, it was first necessary to forge a new and broader definition of the deserving *sick poor* – one that could encompass the new class of patients seeking treatment at the voluntary hospitals.

The sick poor and the new poor

The argument typically advanced today in favour of private social provision, and mimicked in the public sector, is that it empowers the service user through granting them a degree of consumer choice.[7] In the inter-war hospital system it does appear that in some cases ordinary ward patients could upgrade if they could find the money. One woman in Lancashire recalled her sister being offered this option to avoid a waiting list:

> They said it would be twelve months before there were any beds. They asked if she could afford to pay. I said she couldn't really, she just had her hard-earned savings like everybody else. We had been thrifty as we had been fetched up to be thrifty. I asked if she could go somewhere privately. In three days she was in Mount Street Hospital. We didn't choose, they chose. Doesn't that just show? It makes me feel bitter.[8]

Far from empowering working-class patients who *went private*, the memory at least, is of a continuing paternalism governing the voluntary hospitals. For the middle classes it was not a matter of opting to *go private*, as income limits to the ordinary wards ensured private treatment was their only option. Rather, the concern was that those who could afford to pay might try to *go public* by seeking admission to the ordinary wards to save money – something widely seen as an 'abuse' of charity.

Abuse and the diversion of charity

When Dr Thomas Bickerton was writing his medical history of Liverpool, either side of the First World War, he gave considerable prominence to the contemporary issue of 'hospital abuse'. By which he meant 'the exploitation by the unscrupulous and parasitical members of the community of the services' of the voluntary hospitals. 'No one grudged to the destitute the treatment which they received gratuitously at the hospitals and dispensaries', he insisted, 'but it was a grave abuse of charity when those of moderate income expected to receive advice and treatment for which, without hardship, they could afford an adequate fee'. He decried this behaviour as 'the chief form of hospital abuse' and 'disastrous to all concerned'.[9] To demonstrate this, one local report cited the shocking example of a woman 'who openly boasted in the ward that she would have been treated at home if she had not bought a seventy-guinea piano!' [10] This condemnation of those who made unnecessary use of charity was an important moral pillar of late-Victorian paternalism, and one which lived on well into the twentieth century.[11] One almoner who entered the profession in the 1930s recalled this, with a fellow almoner not so much weeding out abuse as defending a patient against the charge:

> I do remember one doctor coming in and saying, 'I'm sure this woman should be a private patient. She's wearing a fur coat', and Margaret Watson, who did know something about this patient, really going at him on the absurdity of assuming that because people wore fur coats, etc, they could manage. The people who weren't clearly hospital patients at that stage were the people with incomes of about £450, the middle class. They could not afford private treatment. They were on the border line of hospital treatment and you had very often to argue that these people should be treated by the hospital and not sent away to Harley Street.[12]

Although this doctor's concerns were shared by the likes of Bickerton, Burdett and the Charity Organisation Society, the initial investigations of newly appointed almoners at London hospitals in late 1890s did not reveal any significant abuse of medical charity. At the Royal Free Hospital, only around 1.5 per cent of outpatients were 'considered able to afford the usual fees for private advice' and were therefore told they would not receive treatment in future.[13] The almoners at St Mary's Hospital also found that the outpatient department had 'not been abused on a large scale', with only 2 per cent being deemed 'unsuitable'.[14] This came as no surprise to some. The governors of Guy's Hospital insisted their outpatient department 'was seldom improperly taken advantage of, and that, with few exceptions, the people attending ... were fit recipients for charitable relief'. The appointment of an almoner provided evidence to support this assertion. Her function was therefore not to stamp out abuse but to serve as a 'pledge' by the governors, 'a further assurance to the public ... of their desire to prevent any abuse'.[15] The moral outrage therefore appears to have been somewhat disproportionate: the middle classes were not a major element of the voluntary hospital patient base at the turn of the century as some feared. Yet those fears were real and they continued into the twentieth century.

Interwar concerns of diverting charitable efforts away from the sick poor were expressed by Labour politicians and trade unionists – 'we do not want the provision of paying beds to be the means of cutting down services for poor people' – and were also found in the hospitals themselves.[16] By 1927 the St John's (skin) Hospital in London had ended its private provision, having found 'there was occasionally a little difficulty with the patients as, naturally, they required more personal attention and the Staff was not large enough to give such extra attention'.[17] Similarly, one interwar GP found the different expectations of his working-class and middle-class patients required him to spend twice as long with the latter.[18] Equally, at the West End Hospital for Nervous Diseases they had found it 'undesirable, both from the Hospital's and the patients' points of view, to have "Hospital" and "part-paying" or "semi-private" patients in close proximity to each other'.[19] Such a statement suggests there may have been some merit to one Scottish MP's concerns that the preferential treatment of private patients was in 'danger of creating class distinction and snobbery'.[20] To avoid these difficulties, it was often the case that the establishment of private wards was part of a wider scheme of hospital extension or reconstruction, or room was made for these wards by clearing a floor of the nurses' home, a part of the hospital site not being used for the treatment of sick poor.[21]

The typical response to such concerns was for hospital governors and administrators to insist that private wards had the opposite effect. At the Bristol Royal Infirmary it was claimed in 1937 that 'the small profit derived from the private patients helps to maintain the beds in the general wards'.[22] However, beyond such claims there is little evidence in Bristol or elsewhere to support the idea of any redistributive effect of private provision.

Expanding the definition of the 'sick poor'

Those who supported the admission of middle-class private patients – whether administrators within the hospitals, reformers in organisations such as the King's Fund, or supporters in parliament – all adopted a strikingly similar rhetorical strategy. This involved an enlarged redefinition, rather than an abandonment, of the notion of the *sick poor*. This term was commonly used by doctors and administrators in interwar hospitals to mean anyone who could not afford the private fees of being treated in their own home. After the First World War major changes of two kinds – advances in medical technology and broader economic changes – brought significantly more people into that category. Technological change meant the hospital could deliver something beyond even the most expensive care at home.[23] This reasoning could easily have been used to support the idea that the modern hospital could no longer be a site for the medical care of the poor exclusively, but rather that it must be a resource for all classes.

This line of argument seems to have had some purchase in the municipal sector. Indeed, two emergent principles of healthcare were promoted by Section 13 of Health Minister Neville Chamberlain's 1929 Local Government Act. One was universalism, by means of granting local authorities the power (if securing Ministry of Health approval) to appropriate poor law infirmaries in order to provide general hospital services to the community as a whole. Meanwhile, co-ordination across the mixed economy was also promoted by stating that there should be consultation with the local voluntary hospitals on such developments.[24] Although not all local authorities took up this opportunity Bristol did, making the appropriation of Southmead Hospital a flagship policy. To some extent this was a matter of reinforcing an established commitment: 'Some time ago', the city's medical officer of health declared in 1930, 'the Board of Guardians opened the doors of Southmead for the treatment of sick persons of all classes.' [25] Yet we also know ordinary and private patients were treated in different wards and paid different amounts.[26] If other areas went further in adopting a universalist approach, Bristol did not join them.

In the voluntary hospitals there was no such change. They did not abandon philanthropy as their organising principle. What did change, or at least what reformers sought to change, was who was seen as a deserving recipient of medical charity. A 1923 Court of Chancery ruling had established the precedent 'that a hospital for "poor" persons could provide pay beds' because they defined the poor as 'persons unable to afford [the] full cost of private treatment', which it estimated at a rather high five guineas.[27] This could therefore include patients drawn from 'the blackcoated poor of the middle and professional classes', with incomes too high to gain admission to the ordinary wards or to receive financial assistance from national insurance, but for whom meeting the costs associated with illness and treatment was still a challenge.[28] Lord Castlerosse wrote in the *Sunday Express* in 1927 that 'this class suffers in the same way as Farmers do, from not combining together in their own interests'.[29] He supported the conclusion of a report by H.L. Eason that the solution lay in middle-class insurance. Yet Eason did not see this being achieved simply by insurance schemes to cover treatment in the odd private bed: 'Until private hospitals are built for this purpose, it will still remain the truth that in England the only people who get properly treated are the rich and the poor, while those of limited means have to put up with an inferior service.'[30] Although the transition was more timid, this echoes the situation whereby the American hospitals 'had gone from treating the poor for the sake of charity to treating the rich for the sake of revenue and only belatedly given thought to the people in between'.[31] Meanwhile the less radical Lord Macmillan, chairman of the Voluntary Hospitals' Parliamentary Committee, insisted it was a philanthropic principle of the established hospitals 'that nobody should be unable to benefit merely because he is embarrassed with regard to money'.[32]

A notable voice making the case that private wards catered for this unfortunate group was the King's Fund. Founded by Henry Burdett in 1897 as the Prince of Wales Hospital Fund for London, it was established to encourage both donations from the middle and upper classes and support the modernisation of the hospitals. This meant introducing the latest systems of accountancy, greater co-ordination between institutions and, increasingly in the interwar years, making provision for private patients.[33] The King's Fund was behind legislation passed in 1936 making it considerably easier for private wards to be introduced at the minority of older hospitals whose trust deeds explicitly referred to catering exclusively for the poor. Where before it took an Act of parliament for these hospitals to be able to establish private wards, afterwards it required only the approval of the Charity Commissioner. In their confidential briefing for the promoters of the Bill, discussed in the previous chapter, the King's Fund presented a picture of private provision somewhat at odds with other evidence now available – one in which private wards were common and the rate of charges was low.[34] Payment, they were implying, was not crowding out philanthropy.

The rhetorical and political strategies adopted by advocates of private provision were based on the premise that middle-class patients needed to be brought in to a revised notion of the sick poor. The arguments of both supporters and opponents rested on the assumption that the traditional mission of the voluntary hospitals – understood to be both philanthropic and paternalistic in character – remained essentially unchanged. Indeed, on the ground we see this embodied in arrangements designed to ensure that, even when middle-class patients were treated, it was not on the same terms as working-class patients. The guiding principle of middle-class exclusion gave way to what we might term *class differentiation*.

Class differentiation

The inclusion of middle-class patients fell far short of heralding the advent of some version of social democratic citizenship in the hospital wards. As early as the 1870s, Burdett sought to legitimise middle-class treatment by separating it from that for the sick poor. He proposed separate private hospitals, beds or wards, operating on a commercial basis, while the working classes would remain as the only patients in the ordinary wards.[35] However, instead of receiving 'free' treatment, he envisaged the ordinary wards operating 'a system of small payments, according to the means of the applicant'.[36] What he was advocating was the adoption of two key principles, which we will here term *economic reciprocalism* (to which we will return) and *class differentiation*. The latter involved the separation of patients into two groups – those who could and those who could not afford to pay for medical treatment themselves – with different sites of and terms of treatment for each.

There was some delay, however, before such ideas were put into practice. Following the 1891 investigation of a House of Lords committee into the over-crowding of voluntary hospital outpatient departments, the Royal Free Hospital in London sought to reassert their focus on treating the sick poor. In order to do so, they appointed an Enquiry Officer, who was quickly replaced by Miss Mary Stewart, a St Pancras social worker employed by the Charity Organisation Society.[37] Thereafter, Stewart trained future almoners for her own and other hospitals before the task was taken over by the COS.[38] With the arrival of the almoner the hospitals had someone who could put into practice this separation of the classes, leaving only the matter of where to draw the dividing line to be settled.

Drawing the line

Initially it appears that Mary Stewart simply used the COS categorisations of applicants for charitable assistance: those who could afford to join a provident association, those unable to afford such payments, and those in need of non-medical assistance.[39] Thus, from the beginning the separation was entirely financial, relating to those who could or could not afford to pay for treatment. By the mid-1920s, this had become standard practice and the BMA suggested where the income limits for ordinary ward treatment might be drawn (see table 5.1). The BMA recommended progressive limits of between £200 and £300 annual income, depending on the size of the dependent family.[40] Corresponding income limits were a feature of the hospital contributory schemes. Indeed, amidst local contributory scheme tensions in 1942, the Bristol Royal Hospital (the merged Royal Infirmary and General Hospital) was said to be insisting upon making enquiries into the circumstances of patients even when they were members of a contributory scheme, if that scheme had not 'given a written pledge to observe the BMA scale of income limits.'[41]

A major study of the contributory scheme movement suggested that Bristol's income limit, set at £312 per annum (or £6 per week), was typical.[42] On average this covered 84 per cent of those living in English county boroughs, but inevitably a little less in Bristol as the city had a large middle-class population. Charles Madge, co-founder of the Mass Observation movement, surveyed Bristol in 1940 and found 81.8 per cent to have incomes below £7.[43] The same dividing

Table 5.1 BMA recommendations for income limits, *c.*1926

Class	Limit	Open to
1	£200	(a) single persons over 16 years of age (b) widow or widower without children under 16 years of age
2	£250	(a) married couples without children under 16 years of age (b) persons with one dependent under 16 years of age
3	£300	(a) married couples with a child or children under 16 years of age (b) persons with more than one dependent under 16 years of age

Source: BSC, DM980 (30), Bristol Hospitals Commission 1941, BHF evidence, appendix 1.

line had been drawn by Henry Tout in his 1937 social survey of the city, which was 'concerned only with incomes which fall below middle-class levels', which he said was 'four-fifths of all Bristol families.'[44] These clear class divisions, drawn according to income levels, were therefore not only evident in social comment but also in the administering of statutory welfare and the mechanics of admission to the city's voluntary hospitals and membership of its hospital contributory schemes. This system of class differentiation meant that different services were provided on different terms to different sections of society.

However, some caveat should be offered to the idea there was a simple means test separating working-class and middle-class patients. Steven Cherry has identified a 'gradation' in rates of payment, though the relationship between this and the separation of the classes has gone uncommented upon.[45] In a 1935 meeting between the King's Fund and the Ministry of Health, Lord Luke explained:

> there was an unbroken gradation, in rates of pay and in accommodation, from ordinary patients paying nothing and ordinary patients paying voluntarily, through patients of limited means paying charges under contract in special part pay beds and patients of moderate means in full pay beds, up to well-to-do patients in expensive beds.[46]

Such a gradation can be seen in the Bristol Royal Infirmary's patient payment scheme, discussed in chapter three. In 1922 there were not only the 15 per cent of patients paying the set amount of twenty-one shillings, the 28 per cent paying various reduced rates and the 55 per cent paying nothing, but also the small 1.5 per cent who paid the set amount plus a donation to the hospital.[47] This suggests a wide gradation, even before the more obvious separation of working-class and middle-class patients with the arrival of private wards later in the decade.

This in fact proved to be an issue in the early 1940s, as the BHF found itself out of line with the British Hospital Contributory Schemes Association's policy of bringing about a national flat rate income limit of £420.[48] Evidently gradation was a resilient feature of hospital payment schemes, despite pressure at the national level to simplify practices in favour of a two-tier split. Both the BMICS's middle-class 'section 2' scheme and the BHF's provident scheme provided access to private wards for those over the income limits of £312 per annum.[49] However, the BHF also had an intermediary scheme which created an additional category of those who were narrowly over the income limit for the general wards, having annual incomes between £312 and £420. Those between the two limits did not receive a superior private alternative; rather, they gained access to the same ordinary ward provision, although to do so they had to make a significantly higher contribution through their 6d weekly membership rate, which was twice that of the main scheme.[50] Although there was disagreement over the particulars of the income limits, the principle that those over the limits should make their own provision and all those below them should receive the same service regardless of how much they were able to contribute was not questioned.

The means test in healthcare and welfare

We can identify a similar approach to welfare more generally during this period. Legislation in 1931 introduced a household means test for those receiving unemployment benefits for more than twenty-six weeks. As with the investigations of the almoner, this social enquiry used an assessment of the household as a whole in determining entitlement. The means test was designed 'to ensure that the state's money would not be claimed unnecessarily'.[51] Similarly, the income limits the almoner policed were designed to avoid the 'abuse' of free or subsidised treatment being given to those who could afford to pay for medical attention. In both cases, there were central guidelines but there was discretion in implementation, whether at local authority or institutional level.[52]

The means test was the iconic policy of the National Government for its opponents, who organised marches and street protests throughout the 1930s. Their criticisms were not only that it was intrusive, but that it was unfair to include pensions, savings and the income of other members of the household when judging the financial position of the individual applicant. Derek Fraser has suggested the latter 'heightened family tension, already aggravated by the loss of patriarchal dignity and discipline consequent upon unemployment itself'.[53] The whole-family assessment remained until 1941, when the household means test became a personal one under Churchill's coalition government.[54] It is therefore not surprising that one Glasgow almoner should feel the need to deny that her household investigations 'in any way smacked of the hated Means Test'.[55]

There is a significant difference, however, between the National Government's means test and the hospital almoner's assessment in terms of where the line was drawn. It was the job of the almoner to find, amongst the patients of her hospital, those for whom sickness did not bring with it financial hardship, those who had the disposable income necessary for medical fees. Holding this up alongside Herbert Tout's categorisation of the Bristol working classes in 1937 may shed further light here. Those below the ordinary ward income limits would include not only those described by Tout as being 'in poverty' or having a 'hard struggle', but also 'typical Bristolians', some of whom 'have a small marginal for saving or pleasure if they are frugal', and also those who he considered to be 'very comfortable by the prevailing standards in the classes covered'.[56] The 'classes covered' were those who were both included in his survey of working-class living standards and in the ordinary wards of the voluntary hospitals. Where the means test separated out the very poorest in order to justify public expenditure, the hospitals' income limits were designed instead to exclude the wealthiest.

This difference aside, they were both systems which used income assessments to determine entitlement to services. The assumption behind both was that those considered not poor enough were able to make their own provisions for hard times. Entitlement to voluntary hospital services in this period should therefore be understood as more akin to the 1930s means test than *going private* today. By establishing a system of class differentiation governing access to the voluntary hospitals, a new patient contract was constructed for working-class patients. We now turn to the role in which this cast them.

Economic reciprocalism

Historians have long discussed the essentially subordinate role of the patient as a recipient of medical and other charity.[57] Moral judgements of working-class life were bound up with the idea that patients should reciprocate by demonstrating their virtue, thereby proving themselves 'deserving' of treatment. We see this reflected in Lynsey Cullen's work on the first almoner, Mary Stewart, appointed to London's Royal Free Hospital in 1895. Following a home visit from her, some patients were refused treatment. Miss Stewart's record book recalls one visit on which she found 'the mother very dirty and untidy, and gossiping in the street'. After another, she considered 'the family to bare [*sic*] good character', that they were 'sober and hardworking, but very poor'. Free treatment was refused in the first case and granted in the second.[58]

This case shows the almoner could be a defender of the traditional philanthropic brand of moral reciprocalism, whereby the patient was expected to not transgress certain behavioural codes. However, it was rare for the almoner to suggest individuals be refused treatment, certainly by the time the profession spread beyond the capital. For the most part, the almoner's role was to assess the circumstances of patients and recommend an appropriate level at which they should be asked to contribute financially to the hospital. As we have seen, the arrival of the almoner and the rise of contributory schemes were important changes, and both show the old principle of moral reciprocalism was giving way to a new economic reciprocalism founded on the notion of earning the right to hospital treatment through financial contribution, as a form of what Finlayson called 'citizenship by contribution'.[59]

Contribution as civic duty: rhetoric and reality
This notion of a civic duty to contribute was expressed in a number of ways. It was commonly asserted in general terms as 'the primary duty of every good citizen'.[60] This was a message that placed working-class

contributions within a broader cross-class fundraising strategy. The London example offers a demonstration of this, with two major organisations established by the hospital reformer Henry Burdett. The King's Fund was designed to bring the prestige of the royal family to philanthropic fundraising amongst the middle classes. Meanwhile, the League of Mercy was established a year later in 1898 as an auxiliary of the Fund and intended to raise funds from 'the poorer classes' who, Burdett noted, were least likely to make charitable donations but most likely to use the services of the hospitals.[61] Similarly, contributory schemes in Bristol sought to elicit donations from employers as well as employees, regardless of the fact they would have been charged as private patients if admitted to the hospitals. Promotional material for Bristol's first major contributory scheme in 1933 asked: 'IS YOUR FACTORY AN 100% ONE?' This meant, they explained, that employer, manager and staff should all contribute. 'IF NOT', they asked, 'WHY NOT?' It was the duty of a good employer to make such a contribution.[62] Likewise, the national association defined the key purpose of the schemes as raising funds for the voluntary hospitals 'primarily from wage-earners and their employers.'[63] A similar line was taken during the Sheffield Voluntary Hospitals' Million Pound Appeal in 1938: 'It is not healthy for any community to depend on one or two benefactors to provide the necessary money for its Hospitals; it is the duty of the community as a whole – it is YOUR responsibility.'[64] In rhetoric at least, contribution was seen to be a universal duty.[65]

Membership was sometimes cast as a duty to one's family, as can be seen in figure 5.1. The same approach was taken by Mr Brookhouse Richards, founding president of the BMICS, when he 'suggested to the wives of every wage-earner in the city that they should insist that it was the duty of her husband to her, the children, and himself, to join the contributory scheme, and so abolish all anxiety as to the future in the case of illness.'[66] A decade later, he encouraged membership by appealing to a different conception of civic duty, a wider responsibility to the community as a whole of contributing to the stewardship of local institutions. Speaking in 1935 he declared:

> These great hospitals were founded by the past generation, but what is the present generation doing to maintain them? We know that in our organization and others like it we have 70,000 contributors, but it is computed that at least 40,000 responsible citizens of Bristol do not

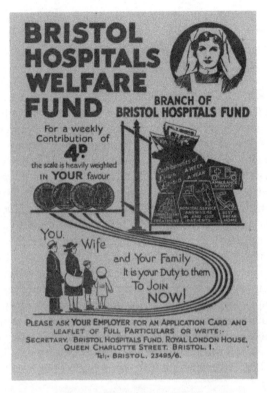

Figure 5.1 Contributory scheme membership depicted as a family
duty, 1943

contribute one penny to voluntary institutions. Yet when the necessity
arises they are the first to seek the privileges of the hospitals, being
enabled to do so through the self-sacrifice of their neighbours ... It is
often said of the people of Bristol that they sleep with one eye open,
I ardently desire them to open the other eye, and take stock of the
unhappy position that some of the hospitals find themselves in to-day,
I would say, Wake up, Bristol, and realize the full extent of your
responsibilities.[67]

Likewise, on the foundation of the BHF, the Bishop of Bristol said the
'alleviation of suffering and the curing of disease is much more than the
responsibility of the religious community. It is the duty of every citizen.'[68]

Meanwhile, contribution was also characterised in BHF promotional material as a personal responsibility, a means for a 'self-respecting citizen' to 'pay their way'.[69] Similar dynamics were evident in Belfast. This was evident when the lord chief justice, Sir Denis Henry, stated during the hospital's annual meeting in 1923 that the subscribers 'did not want to be treated as paupers; they were honest, hard-working men, who were prepared, God helping them, to pay their way'.[70] In the eyes of the hospital's leadership, willingness to make a financial contribution demonstrated deservingness of medical relief.

Evidence that such statements were not just fundraising rhetoric but voiced genuinely held values is clear from the reaction when it was believed patients or schemes had not paid their way. For example, Herbert Baker, president of the Bristol General Hospital, noted in reference to motor crashes that: 'Although some victims were generous, others passing through the city did not pay what they should'.[71] Similarly, there were cases where the reciprocal arrangements between schemes from different areas, so that if people fell ill away from home they would still receive the benefits of contribution, were either not adhered to or deemed inadequate. The BHF had such an arrangement with a Torquay scheme, although the BHF secretary John Dodd described their rate of payment to the Bristol hospitals as 'absolutely absurd'. During the Second World War he commented: 'One would think it impossible for any borough the size of Torquay, even though they have not received much attention from the enemy, to calmly go on as though they have no obligations to their neighbours in these days. I shall certainly tell them what I think of them every time they try and shift their responsibility on to Bristol citizens.'[72]

It is notable that those hospitals in Bristol outside of this system – where their patients were often not categorised as ordinary patients and therefore where contributory schemes were not a factor – did not undergo the same cultural-ideological repositioning. Wholesome behaviour continued to be the primary concern at two hospitals in Bristol. One was the Orthopaedic Hospital and Home for Crippled Children, which received typically less than 2 per cent of ordinary income from contributory schemes.[73] The other was the Bristol Temporary Home and Lying-in Hospital, which was not affected by contributory schemes as they did not cover 'ordinary maternity cases'. It stuck to its commitment 'to exercise a *moral* and *religious* influence over the girls, to help them to regain their own self-respect and that of others'.[74] The continuance of a moralistic premise for admission was reflected in their annual reports which until the 1940s stated the core mission of the institution as being: 'to receive and influence for good young women who are expecting to become mothers for the FIRST time, and who have never mixed with degraded companions; also to place the infants in charge of responsible women, from whose care they cannot be removed without the sanction of the Committee'.[75] In both cases, the role of the patient appears to have been understood in socio-behavioural terms, akin to the old-fashioned moral reciprocalism. It is not possible to say whether the involvement of contributory schemes caused the shift to economic reciprocalism or vice versa, or whether the absence of both in these two institutions was caused by overriding moral concerns relating to children and mothers. What is clear, however, is that the rise of economic reciprocalism came hand-in-hand with the contributory scheme movement.

Contribution and citizenship

Even with these exceptions we can, without entirely displacing the late Victorian 'high point of civic Liberalism', recognise the scope and pen-etration of economic notions of civic duty prevalent in the voluntary hospitals and more widely in the interwar years.[76] While this does imply interwar ideas of civic duty were more expansive than simply voting, the patient contract remained essentially passive.[77] Patients making a financial contribution, even those middle-class patients paying a com-mercial rate, were not empowered medical citizen-consumers of the kind seen since the 1960s.[78] They were understood as *active* citizens only in the sense that they acted upon their obligations to the hospital and to the community. Indeed, the only reason these were common civic duties rather than the responsibilities of the individual patient was because all working-class people, and increasingly the middle classes too, were potential patients. Meanwhile, the universal responsibility to pay in to the system was stronger than any notion of universal right to receive relief in the voluntary hospitals, although this was no longer so clearly the case by the time almoners were emphasising the social work side of their role in anticipation of the rest disappearing with the arrival of the NHS.

Wartime arrangements and the spectre of the welfare state disturbed this pattern and the almoner profession certainly saw its interests best served by realigning with social democratic notions of citizenship. Yet the systems built around older paternalistic attitudes were far from hollowed out ideologically by the advent of the postwar welfare state. Finlayson saw something similar despite the advance of the state in 1930s unemployment relief, where 'the frontier of the state moved, but took voluntarist convictions with it'.[79] This meant public assistance means testing mixed the new financial with the old moral distinctions between deserving and underserving. Meanwhile, voluntary associations continued to play a significant role in social case work with the unemployed. Hulme sees this as 'a partnership, where voluntarism provided the personal moral impetus, and the state acted as the impersonal financial backer'.[80] In the field of hospital care, the handover to the state had been less clean or complete. Consequently, the transfer of responsibility for funding relief had not been one from charity to state but rather one from charity to a diverse range of sources including the patients themselves. The end of distributing funds in one case and the beginning of collecting payments in the other produced, to some extent, the same effect. In both cases the interwar years saw social work in the voluntary sector reinterpreting and reinforcing the old social contract at the heart of philanthropy.

Contribution as insurance: rhetoric and reality

The almoner and payment systems were, therefore, far from empowering ones. As an alternative, membership of a contributory scheme did allow for a degree of control to be taken over the management of that financial contribution to the hospital. The cost could be spread out and the almoner interview, which was undoubtedly 'resented' by some as a 'humiliating' experience, could be avoided.[81] Yet the schemes did not advertise themselves as offering an alternative to the almoner or effectively managing the financial contribution of a good citizen. Instead, despite the fact that membership had no bearing on the right to hospital admission or treatment, the schemes were promoted implicitly, and sometimes explicitly, as a form of medical insurance.

The notion of contributory scheme membership as a type of insurance was only reinforced by the rhetoric that had been present since the foundation of the BMICS. Indeed, the scheme's first president, Mr Brookhouse Richards, had stated its objective, as well as raising funds for the hospitals, as being 'to assist those unable to afford it to have the treatment without burdening themselves, their families, or the hospitals. That was not charity,' he said, 'but pure common sense, which ought to appeal to every thinking man and woman.'[82] Likewise, the Dean of Bristol described the BMICS as 'something to enable the man not so fortunately placed as other men, for some small contribution to take away something that will free his mind of any thought of big expenses, if illness comes along'. He continued: 'Surely this is one of the best forms of insurance that has ever been started.'[83] Both Bristol's major schemes, in fact, promoted themselves implicitly as insurance schemes. The BMICS described membership as 'A First-Class Investment for a Rainy Day!', while the BHF encouraged people to 'anchor' themselves to the organisation for financial security (see figure 5.2).[84] These representations are quite at odds with the more honest depiction of membership fees contributing to the fundraising efforts of the hospitals used only two years later (see figure 3.5).

Key to the fundraising/insurance issue is the question of whether members who had paid into a scheme had earned a 'right' to hospital treatment if taken ill. Quite simply, they had not. However, Martin Gorsky and John Mohan have suggested that contributory schemes 'were perceived by their members as having the character of insurance' and that they had, by virtue of contribution, earned a 'moral right' to treatment.[85] Meanwhile, Barry Doyle has focused on the ways in which such a perceived right might be enforced through working-class representation in hospital governance, identifying hospital contributory schemes as arenas within which power and control could be negotiated.[86] Rather than commercial insurance, this had a strong mutual character, with a 'dual thread of self-interest and humanitarianism.'[87] Indeed, William Beveridge noted approvingly in 1948 that the recent growth of hospital contributory schemes had 'shown the driving force that emerges when local feeling can be combined with Mutual Aid'.[88] Yet it is hard not to reach the conclusion that promoting the schemes as offering insurance was a rather misleading fundraising strategy.

There was some tension here between philanthropy and mutualism – what Beveridge dubbed the 'impulse from above' and the 'impulse

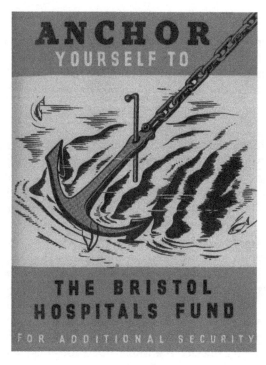

Figure 5.2 Contributory scheme membership depicted as an 'anchor', 1946

from below'[89] – but they were not fundamentally pulling in different directions. Certainly, the early twentieth century did see the growth of the expectation of access to healthcare as a right and contributory schemes were pivotal in this development.[90] Yet in practice they served no function in meeting this expectation for individual patients. As extensions of the hospital administration, the contributory schemes served two key functions. One was raising funds, which they provided both as payments to cover the contribution of their members when admitted and in block grants to support the general work of the institution. The other was to normalise and celebrate working-class financial contributions to the hospitals.

Accepting payment

There is some evidence that the notion of contribution as a civic duty was not just held by those running the contributory schemes and the voluntary hospitals, but amongst the working classes as well – and this is to be found in the membership figures of contributory schemes.

Contributory scheme membership

While criticising the forerunners to his own scheme, John Dodd suggested that the level of membership in Bristol compared poorly with that of other cities. He listed the impressive number of contributors in cities such as Sheffield (250,000), Liverpool (332,000) and Birmingham (600,000) in 1937.[91] He did not, however, offer any membership figure for Bristol. This may have been because of an important difference between Bristol and these other cities. Sheffield, Liverpool and Birmingham all had one single, central scheme. Consequently, the membership of that scheme was in itself the total membership for the city. In Bristol, the BMICS was a central scheme operating alongside a great many smaller local and workplace schemes, while Dodd's BHF was set up as yet another scheme largely in an effort to unify the myriad schemes operating in the city. It was therefore much harder to give a reliable figure for the city as a whole. Some rough figure can be estimated from combining the stated membership figures of the Bristol Hospital Contributors League,[92] which brought together the BMICS and the smaller schemes, with the published membership rates of the BHF.[93] This suggests that contributory scheme membership in Bristol in the early 1940s was in the region of 150,000. Certainly this is less than those of some other major English provincial cities, but compares well with the nearby cities of South Wales. Swansea's was the largest scheme in Wales with 114,000 members in 1941, while Cardiff's had only 66,000.[94] Bristol's contributory scheme membership rate may not have been amongst the highest, therefore, but it can hardly be considered low.

Charles Madge's analysis of Tout's 1937 Bristol survey suggests that a majority of working-class families were making a contribution.[95] Some 62.4 per cent of all working-class families were said to contribute to hospital funds, and amongst families headed by skilled and semi-skilled male labourers, who might be considered the respectable working classes, the percentage rose to 74.3 and 78.5 respectively.[96] We can safely assume these rates increased once we include the new contributors signed up to the BHF, established two years later, even if some were previously contributors to other schemes. Such membership rates amongst the city's working classes demonstrate a widespread acceptance of contribution as a civic duty, especially given the extensive exemptions from general ward payments for those on low incomes that ensured membership was not the only way to receive treatment without paying. Yet we cannot assume that everyone who joined a contributory scheme supported or agreed with the principle of economic reciprocalism. There are various other reasons why individuals may have joined.

An oral history informant described the establishment of the one-penny-per-week employees' hospital scheme at Storeys' mill in Lancaster: 'You might call it voluntary because in the first place they might have called a meeting of the workers: "Have you any objections to one penny being deducted from your wage?" Then it was automatic, that was that … If you paid you did [get free treatment] and if you couldn't you couldn't.'[97] We can also assume that some people joined contributory schemes out of a mistaken belief, encouraged by the schemes' promotion, that they would be buying some otherwise unavailable guarantee of access when sick as a form of insurance. Indeed, it was a complaint at the London-based HSA, the largest contributory scheme, that they were often referred to mistakenly as the *Hospital Savings Association* rather than the *Hospital Saving Association*.[98] However, given the scale of almoner reductions and exemptions, it is simply not credible to think that all those who contributed did so mistakenly. Meanwhile, if the arrangements were widely understood but also widely resented, we could expect to see some evidence of resistance or protest.

Alternatively, there may also have been some financial sense in membership for those who were not on a low enough income to be passed free, but still below the income limits. It is worth remembering that the standard charge (although only asked of a minority of assessed patients) was one guinea for a week's stay. At a common rate of 3d per week membership fee it would take over a year and a half (eighty-four weeks) for membership subscriptions to cost the same. Meanwhile, we should not dismiss the pride taken in effective management of a household budget.[99] These positive explanations are more convincing than

the assumption that millions of working people failed to understand
what would happen if they went to hospital and were consequently
duped.

Insurance normalised

It may be that such a view found easy acceptance because it felt familiar.
After all, the principle of paying in to the health and welfare system you
rely on also ran through both the mutual aid societies of the day and
the National Insurance system established by Lloyd George in 1911.
Indeed, with hospital treatment omitted from National Insurance provisions, the contributory schemes could be seen as a complementary
part of the same welfare arrangements. This is not to say they were
insurance schemes. Rather, in their respective areas, there was a shared
premise between what we are here calling *economic reciprocalism*
and the Liberal *insurance principle*. One of Lloyd George's chief civil
servants summarised this when he said 'working people ought to pay
something! It gave them a feeling of self-respect and what cost nothing
was not valued'.[100] That said, pragmatic motivations also prompted the
development of both, with financial pressures paramount for the hospitals and politics playing no small part in guiding the choices of the
Liberal reformers.[101]

The insurance principle, however, was not universally accepted.
Writing at the time, Hilaire Belloc claimed that the 1911 Act, with its
class-based interference, followed 'in every particular the lines of a
Servile State'.[102] He represented a significant block of opinion when,
objecting to its compulsion, he termed it a 'vile enslaving act'.[103] Despite
such criticisms, Lloyd George's judgement was that using insurance as
the premise for his scheme made it socially acceptable and paying insurance came to be treated as any other household expense.[104] A Ministry
of Labour inquiry found that the combined payments of state and voluntary insurance accounted for over 5 per cent of expenditure in the
average working-class household in 1937–38 (see table 5.2). That on
state insurance was 2s 0¾d, while that on voluntary insurance higher
still at 2s 4½d, and an additional 1s 8d was spent on 'medical fees, drugs
and hospitals'.[105] With the insurance principle ingrained, not only as
part of statutory and voluntary welfare systems, but also as part of the
household budget, it is perhaps not surprising that such an attitude
towards voluntary hospital services should develop.

Table 5.2 Average weekly working-class household expenditure, 1937–38

Item	s.	d.	%
Food	34	1	40.1
Rent	10	10	12.7
Clothing	8	2	9.6
Fuel and light	6	5	7.5
Insurance (state and voluntary)	4	5¼	5.2
Household equipment (utensils, etc.)	4	1	4.8
Tobacco and cigarettes	2	6½	3.0
Fares	2	3	2.6
Medical fees, drugs and hospitals	1	8	2.0
Trade Union subscriptions	1	4½	1.6
Cinemas, theatres, football matches, etc.	1	4½	1.6
Newspapers and periodicals	1	0	1.2
Other	6	10¼	8.1
Total	*85*	*1*	*100*

Source: Mark Abrams, *The Condition of the British People 1911–1945* (London, 1946), pp. 84–5.

Considering the impact of such an approach, both parallels and divergence can be seen between National Insurance and the economic reciprocalism of the voluntary hospitals. Lloyd George had an amendment inserted into the 1911 Bill stating 'that medical treatment shall be given without regard to cause or nature of disease', which Derek Fraser used as evidence that he and Churchill 'saw no place in insurance for the concept of the undeserving poor', but instead saw 'universal entitlement earned by contribution.'[106] Likewise, there was no notion of an *undeserving* contributory scheme member, but that is not to say they operated on the same insurance principle. Payment, either directly by the patient or indirectly via a contributory scheme, was in effect an act of good citizenship rather than earning the right to treatment. Moreover, for many Liberal reformers, including Churchill and Beveridge, an important characteristic of the National Insurance scheme was run on an actuarial basis: entitlements were earned by virtue of payment and they were limited accordingly.[107]

For an actuarial approach to be adopted by the voluntary hospitals, they would have had to make payment a condition of access, and this (at least for the ordinary wards) did not happen. However, the deservingness of the individual to receive treatment did move away from moral judgements in favour of three criteria: that they should be in medical need, that they should be unable to pay for the necessary treatment privately, and that they be prepared to make whatever contribution (perhaps none) was deemed appropriate. What the hospitals were operating therefore was closer to the practice Steven Thompson has found amongst the mutualistic welfare provisions of the South Wales Miners' Federation. Although 'membership conferred rights of eligibility' for their various welfare services, 'strict actuarial insurance principles' were rejected in favour of responding wherever possible to the greatest need.[108] This, again, is evidence of the overriding and continuing commitment to the philanthropic traditionalism at the heart of the patient contract in the voluntary hospitals.

Payment and professional identity

In his famous study on Victorian *Outcast London*, Gareth Stedman Jones identified what he called 'the deformation of the gift'. By this he meant that the reciprocity at the heart of philanthropy's meeting of rich and poor was in danger if the interaction was depersonalised; for example, by the geographical separation of the classes through suburbanisation.[109] Such concerns hovered over the hospital in the interwar years, less as a result of another wave of suburbanisation than as a consequence of the broadening patient base. In combating this, the almoner was a powerful figure – policing this system and promoting the principle of economic reciprocalism. Yet in doing so she appears an almost anachronistic figure. Theories of governance tell us authority in this period was diffuse, leading to the working classes being 'steered' towards good civic behaviours rather than old-fashioned Victorian-style 'social control' being exerted.[110] Indeed, we might see something of this in the new style of community activity, especially that geared towards fundraising, that Nick Hayes and Barry Doyle have identified as part of an evolving hospital-orientated middle-class civic culture in the interwar years.[111] While the distinction between the two is at best hazy, the almoner's 'steering' of working-class patients was somewhat heavy-handed for this narrative. Yet the almoner's assessment is an instructive social encounter specific to the interwar years, a ritual that gives us an unusual insight into what Tom Hulme calls 'the actual mechanics of producing citizens'.[112]

The work of producing citizens was an important role for the hospital and carried great influence over the patient as a recipient of medical charity. But it was also a crucial role in building the professional status and identity of the almoner. Where our focus has been on what it meant to *make* a payment or to be *asked* to make one, it is also important to briefly consider the professional meaning of *taking* or *refusing* a payment. Indeed, the rationale for the almoner not only collecting payments but also setting their rate was that she had some specialist insight. It was her training, skill, and experience which allowed her to understand not only the social conditions of the patient but also the wider health and welfare systems to which they might turn for support. This was what allowed her to make a judgement on what was an appropriate level of payment.[113] By the same logic, the almoner could demonstrate professional ability by labelling a patient 'unable to pay' or even refusing a payment offered – showing she had a fine enough appreciation of family circumstances to know when the money was needed at home.[114] Meanwhile, providing free treatment to the poor was a professional activity doctors traded on lucratively in their private practice.[115] In either case, refusal of payment could enhance professional status.

In between taking and refusing payment, a profession might *distance* itself from the payment taken. Indeed, that was essentially what the medical staffs of the hospitals were doing when almoners were brought in to conduct this work. For general practitioners visiting working-class homes, it had long been the 'unwritten law' that after the doctoring had finished a sixpence would be placed on the corner of the table and picked up on the way out.[116] Finding ways to similarly keep doctoring and taking payment separate was not only a question of maintaining the traditional doctor–patient relationship, although this was certainly a factor. It was also one of managing the philanthropic conduct of the institution. We see this when almoners joined doctors in insisting on another third party to collect fees from private patients – those for medical services rather than hospital accommodation. Physicians and surgeons having to collect their own fees was a source of great dissatisfaction following the introduction of private beds at the Bristol Royal

Infirmary in 1926 – a situation only resolved six years later by 'the Secretary's kind offer to collect fees on their behalf.'[117] Moreover, it was an important condition that these fees were not passed on to the individual physician or surgeon, but placed into a collective staff fund, further distancing the doctor from the payment made to them.[118]

For almoners, the collecting of payment in the large working-class wards was often a task undertaken jointly with clerks or administrative assistants.[119] This could have served doubly to enhance professional standing by distancing from the actual collection and by putting on show their seniority over other, often male, colleagues. Where almoners were involved in collecting payments from private patients, however, this tended to be the task of the almoner herself. A 1947 questionnaire from the Institute of Almoners, responded to by 233 hospitals, found 0.5 per cent of almoner's departments collecting medical fees from private patients and none being assisted in doing so. When it came to collecting maintenance fees from private patients, almoners were much more likely to be involved. Fourteen per cent of departments collected those fees, with 9.5 per cent saying this was done by the almoner, 2.5 per cent a clerk and 2 per cent an administrative assistant.[120] Given the limited scale of private provision in the voluntary hospitals, discussed in the previous chapter, this level of activity is considerable.

The eagerness for the almoner profession to abandon this aspect of their work was evident when various charges were introduced only a few years after the establishment of the National Health Service. Under Attlee's Labour government these began with charges for dentures and spectacles, and the door was opened for Churchill's subsequent Conservative government to bring in charges for prescriptions and hospital appliances. Just as the medical staff of the voluntary hospitals had been weary of directly receiving payments, for fear of sullying their hands with the dirty business of money, the almoners were adamant they would not – as some hospital administrators planned – be collecting these new charges. In February 1952, the council of the Institute of Almoners met and issued a statement declaring: 'THAT ANY ASSESSMENT OR COLLECTION OF CHARGES UNDER THE NATIONAL HEALTH SERVICE IS NOT AN APPROPRIATE DUTY OF ALMONERS' DEPARTMENTS AND IN NO CIRCUMSTANCES SHOULD ALMONERS (OR THEIR CLERKS) ACCEPT SUCH RESPONSIBILITIES.'[121]

Refusal to return to their traditional role in assessing patients also meant they sought to have no role in 'dealing with cases of hardship', which they saw as the business of the new National Assistance Board. In rejecting such tasks, the almoners saw themselves as fighting off a distraction from and a dilution of their real work. At their national association's annual general meeting shortly after, Miss Hornsby Smith remarked: 'I am sure many of you rejoice in the fact that your work is no longer association with the extraction of money and that those other services which you render to the patient and to the National Health Service have assumed their proper place.' [122] This was not merely protestation from the social workers. A month later Ministry of Health officials were stating in no uncertain terms that despite the new charges there was no be 'no requirement whatsoever for any person in the almoner's department to assess need' and that there was no suggestion 'that the almoner should be responsible for the collection of money'.[123]

Conclusions

In the summer of 1948, every household in Britain received a leaflet introducing them to *The New National Health Service*. The services of which they were entitled to, free at the point of use, as a right of citizenship: 'There are no charges, except for a few special items. There are no insurance qualifications. But it is not a charity. You are all paying for it, mainly as taxpayers, and it will relieve your money worries in times of illness.'[124] This philosophy was expressed in similar terms by the Prime Minister, Clement Attlee, in a Home Service broadcast on the evening before the 'appointed day' when the NHS and a number of other Labour reforms came into effect. The NHS would, he said, give 'a complete cover for health by pooling the nation's resources and paying the bill collectively'. However, this was not a state-run social insurance scheme: 'It is not dependent on insurance, everyone is eligible'. Rather, healthcare had become a nationalised industry.[125]

This was not only a break in who provided healthcare, but also in its underlying philosophy of citizenship. Attlee and Bevan alike were keen to emphasise that entitlement to NHS services was neither insurance nor charity. By contrast, entitlement to treatment for the pre-NHS citizen patient was understood as both. The meaning of *paying in* to the hospital, either in advance through a mutualist scheme or directly when admitted, was to make a financial contribution. For the majority with working-class levels of income, admission was not dependent on payment but on medical need. To receive that treatment without making what payment was deemed appropriate would have been shameful. For the most part, therefore, patient payments were a mediated form of charitable donation.

This was different for that far smaller number of middle-class patients, for whom payment was a commercial arrangement and a necessity to receive treatment. Above all, it is the difference between the two that is telling. The very fact private patients were separate and treated differently tells us that, for all the changes, the main business of the hospitals was still understood in the same terms. The old social divisions and distinctions survived, even as they were brought within the hospital.

Notes

1 See for example Brian Abel-Smith, *The Hospitals 1800–1948* (London: Heinemann, 1964), p. 338; John Pickstone, *Medicine and Industrial Society: A History of Hospital Development in Manchester and Its Region* (Manchester: Manchester University Press, 1985), p. 259; Stephen Cherry, 'Hospital Saturday, Workplace Collections and Issues in Late Nineteenth-Century Hospital Funding', *Medical History*, 44:4 (2000), 462; Steven Cherry, 'Beyond National Health Insurance. The Voluntary Hospitals and Hospital Contributory Schemes: A Regional Study', *Social History of Medicine*, 5:3 (1992), 455.

2 For a classic expression of this expectation see Karl Polanyi, *The Great Transformation*, 1957 edition (Boston: Beacon Press, 1944), p. 57.

3 For a good introduction to the literature in this area, see Marion Foucade and Kieran Healey, 'Moral Views of Market Society', *Annual Review of Sociology*, 33 (2007), 285–311.

4 See Martin Gorsky, ' "For the Treatment of Sick Persons of All Classes": The Transformation of Bristol's Hospital Services, 1918–1939' in Peter Wardley (ed.), *Bristol Historical Resource*, CD-ROM (Bristol: University of the West of England, 2001); and Barry M. Doyle, 'Competition and Cooperation in Hospital Provision in Middlesbrough, 1918–1948', *Medical History*, 51:3 (2007), 337–56.

5 See for example M.J.D. Roberts, *Making English Morals: Voluntary Association and Moral Reform in England, 1787–1886* (Cambridge: Cambridge University Press, 2004).

6 For a similar trend identified in nineteenth-century Birmingham, see Jonathan Reinarz, 'Investigating the "Deserving" Poor: Charity, Discipline and Voluntary Hospitals in Nineteenth-Century Birmingham' in Peter Shapely and Anne Borsay (eds), *Medicine, Charity and Mutual Aid: The Consumption of Health and Welfare, c.1550–1950* (Aldershot: Ashgate, 2006).

7 See, for example, Natalie Arend, Dan Corry, Warren Hatter, Julian Le Grand and Adam Lent, *Choice: What Role Can It Play in Helping Local Public Services Evolve?* (London: New Local Government Network, 2003).

8 Lucinda McCray Beier, *For Their Own Good: The Transformation of English Working-Class Health Culture, 1880–1970* (Columbus: Ohio State University Press, 2008), p. 135.

9 Thomas H. Bickerton, *A Medical History of Liverpool from the Earliest Days to the Year 1920* (London: J. Murray, 1936), p. 251.

10 *Ibid.*, p. 253.

11 On late Victorian concern about abuse, see Keir Waddington, 'Unsuitable Cases: The Debate over Outpatient Admissions, the Medical Profession and Late-Victorian London Hospitals', *Medical History*, 42:1 (1998), 26–46.

12 MRC, Jean Snelling, Social Workers Speak Out, 1980, p. 10, http://www2.warwick.ac.uk/services/library/mrc/explorefurther/speakingarchives/socialwork/929.publ_no_18_j_snelling.pdf, accessed 25 April 2016.

13 MRC, MSS.378/IMSW/A/1/1/4: 'Extract from Hospital reports re enquiry. Royal Free.' 1897.

14 335 out of 12,562 outpatients. MSS.378/IMSW/A/1/1/4: 'Extract from Hospital reports re enquiry. St Mary's.' 1897.

15 A total of 52 out of 6,288 outpatients were 'refused treatment on the grounds of not being proper subjects for charitable relief' in the almoner's first year. MRC, MSS.378/IMSW/A/1/1/4: 'Extract from Hospital reports re enquiry. Guy's.' 1897.

16 Lord Sanderson, HL Deb 2 April 1935, vol. 96, cc. 467–8.

17 LMA, A/KE/166, King's Fund, completed questionnaires from hospitals without pay beds but having schemes for providing them, 1927. See also Robert Dingwall, Anne Marie Rafferty, and Charles Webster, *An Introduction to the Social History of Nursing* (London: Routledge, 1988), pp. 74–5.

18 Wellcome Collection, CMAC 29/1/71, Interview with Eric Grogono cited in Anne Digby, *The Evolution of British General Practice, 1850–1948* (Oxford: Oxford University Press, 1999), p. 240.

19 LMA, A/KE/166, King's Fund, completed questionnaires from hospitals without pay beds but having schemes for providing them, 1927. The category of 'part-paying' or 'semi-private' patients appears to refer to those middle-class patients sharing a room with another patient and paying less than those in single rooms.

20 Mr Mathers, HC Deb 8 May 1936, vol. 311, c. 2050.

21 For St Bartholomew's Hospital see LMA, A/KE/166, King's Fund, completed questionnaires from hospitals without pay beds but having schemes for providing them, 1927. For Sheffield see TNA, MH 58/319, Precis of Memorandum dated 5 April 1938, prepared by the Honorary Staffs of the Voluntary Hospitals for Presentation to the 'Sheffield Municipal and Voluntary Advisory Committee', p. 4.

22 BRI, *Report for 1937*, p. 16.

23 For a contemporary comment on this and its implication for the provision of health services, see Ministry of Health, Consultative Council on Medical and Allied Services, *Interim Report on the Future Provision of Medical and Allied Services* (London: HMSO, 1920), p. 5.

24 Alysa Levene, Martin Powell, and John Stewart, 'Patterns of Municipal Health Expenditure in Interwar England and Wales', *Bulletin of the History of Medicine*, 78:3 (2004), 644–6; John Mohan and Martin Gorsky, *Don't Look Back? Voluntary and Charitable Finance of Hospital in Britain, Past and Present* (London: Office of Health Economics & Association of Chartered Certified Accountants, 2001), p. 38; David Owen, *English Philanthropy 1660–1960* (Cambridge, MA: Harvard University Press, 1966), p. 502.

25 BRO, Health Committee Minutes, 1 Jan 1930.

26 TNA, MH 66/1068, 'County Borough of Bristol' by Allan C Parsons (Ministry of Health, 1932), p. 142; Almoner's Reports in Bristol Medical Officer of Health Reports for 1937 and 1938.

27 LMA, A/KE/185, King's Fund, memorandum etc on paying patients in hospitals, 1934–1936.

28 Lord Luke, HL Deb 10 December 1935, vol. 99, c. 128; and 2 April 1935, vol. 96, c. 466. This might also include the cost of care in a nursing home: Viscount Hailsham, HL Deb 2 April 1935, vol. 96, c. 476.

29 Lord Castlerosse, 'Middle Class Muddle', *Sunday Express*, 20 November 1927 (see LMA, A/KE/169).

30 Eason quoted in Castlerosse, 'Muddle'.

31 Paul Starr, *The Social Transformation of American Medicine* (New York: Basic Books, 1982), p. 159.

32 Lord Macmillan, HL Deb 2 April 1935, vol. 96, cc. 479–80.

33 For more on the history of the King's Fund see F.K. Prochaska, *Philan-thropy and the Hospitals of London: The King's Fund, 1897–1990* (Oxford: Clarendon Press, 1992).

34 LMA, A/KE/185, King's Fund, VHPPB, Information for Promoters (con-fidential), 27 March 1935. It is unclear how the remaining 172 beds were categorised.

35 Henry Burdett, *Pay Hospitals and Paying Wards throughout the World: Facts in Support of a Re-Arrangement of the English System of Medical Relief* (London: J.&A. Churchill, 1879), p. 30.

36 *Ibid.*, p. 21.

37 Moberley Bell, Enid, *The Story of the Hospital Almoners: The Birth of a Profession* (London: Faber & Faber, 1961), p. 27.

38 Lynsey Cullen, 'The First Lady Almoner: The Appointment, Position, and Findings of Miss Mary Stewart at the Royal Free Hospital, 1895–99', *Journal of the History of Medicine and Allied Sciences*, 68:4 (2013), 562.

39 Almoners Report Book, Royal Free Hospital Archives, RFH/6/A/1, p.8, cited in Cullen, 'Almoner', p. 570.

40 BSC, DM980 (30), Bristol Hospitals Commission, BHF evidence, appen-dix 1.

41 BSC, DM980 (28), Letter from Mr Dodd of BHF to Mr Hyde of NPHT, 23 June 1942.

42 Martin Gorsky, John Mohan and Tim Willis, *Mutualism and Health Care: British Hospital Contributory Schemes in the Twentieth Century* (Manches-ter: Manchester University Press, 2006), p. 74; BSC, DM980 (5), Bristol & District Divisional Hospitals Council, Report on Standing Committee meeting on the impact of the 1941 National Health Insurance Contribu-tory Pensions and Workmen's Compensation Act, 30 January 1942 [here-after NHI Report].

43 Charles Madge, 'The Propensity to Save in Blackburn and Bristol', *Eco-nomic Journal*, 50:200 (1940), 411.

44 Herbert Tout, *The Standard of Living in Bristol* (Bristol: University of Bristol: Arroswmith, 1938), p. 11.

45 Steven Cherry, 'Accountability, Entitlement, and Control Issues and Vol-untary Hospital Funding c.1860–1939', *Social History of Medicine*, 9:2 (1996), 215–33.

46 LMA, A/KE/185, Lord Luke in minutes of meeting, April 1935.

47 BRI, *Report for 1922*, p. 21.

48 BSC, DM980 (12), Bristol & District Divisional Hospitals Council, Income Limits Committee Minutes, 27 August 1943.

49 BSC, DM980 (5), Bristol & District Divisional Hospitals Council, Standing Committee, agenda and notes, 31 December 1945; and NHI Report.

50 BSC, DM980 (12), Bristol & District Divisional Hospitals Council, Income Limits Committee Minutes, 27 August 1943; and NHI Report.

51 Stephanie Ward, 'The Means Test and the Unemployed in South Wales and the North-East of England, 1931–1939', *Labour History Review*, 74:1 (2008), 144.

52 *Ibid.*

53 Derek Fraser, *The Evolution of the British Welfare State: A History of Social Policy since the Industrial Revolution*, 3rd edition (Basingstoke: Palgrave Macmillan, 2003), p. 211.

54 Ronald Davison, 'Britain Abolishes the Household Means Test', *Social Service Review*, 15:1 (1941), 534.

55 D.A. Dow, M.M. Leitch and A.F. MacLean, *From Almoner to Social Worker: Social Work at Glasgow Royal Infirmary, 1932–1982* (Glasgow: Glasgow Royal Infirmary, 1982), p. 10.

56 Tout, *Standard of Living*, p. 11.

57 For example, see Roy Porter, 'The Gift Relation: Philanthropy and Provincial Hospitals in Eighteenth-Century England' in Lindsay Granshaw and Roy Porter (eds), *The Hospital in History* (London: Routledge, 1989), p. 150; Colin Jones, 'Some Recent Trends in the History of Charity', in Martin Daunton (ed.), *Charity, Self-Interest and Welfare in the English Past* (London: UCL Press, 1996), pp. 51–63; Alan Kidd, 'Philanthropy and the "Social History Paradigm"', *Social History*, 2:2 (1996), 184 and 186–7; Mary Fissell, *Patients, Power, and the Poor in Eighteenth-Century Bristol* (Cambridge: Cambridge University Press, 1991), pp. 11 and 196–7.

58 Royal Free Hospital Archives, RFH/6/A/1, Almoner's Record Book, pp. 17–19. For further discussion of Mary Stewart, see Cullen, 'Almoner'.

59 See Geoffrey Finlayson, *Citizen, State, and Social Welfare in Britain 1830–1990* (Oxford: Oxford University Press, 1994), p. 9 and *passim*.

60 BMICS, *Report for 1931*, p. 8.

61 Prochaska, *King's Fund*, p. 35; Frank Prochaska, 'Burdett, Sir Henry Charles (1847–1920)', *Oxford Dictionary of National Biography*, Oxford: Oxford University Press, 2004, http://0-www.oxforddnb.com. pugwash.lib.warwick.ac.uk/view/article/38827, accessed 25 April 2016.

62 BMICS, *Report for 1933*, inside back cover.

63 BCWA, Extracts from BHCSA points of policy for hospital contributory schemes, 1937.

64 Sheffield United Hospitals Collection, Printed Brochure, 'Sheffield Voluntary Hospitals Million Pound Appeal', The City Hall, Tuesday, 19 July

1938, SCA NHS12/3/6/3, cited in Barry Doyle, *The Politics of Hospital Provision in Early 20th-Century Britain* (London: Pickering & Chatto, 2014), p. 130.

65   BMICS, *Report for 1931*, p. 8; BSC, DM980, (4), Bristol & District Divisional Hospitals Council, Chairman's File, no.1, Alderman Burgess' notes on Report of the Aero Engines Ltd Welfare Superintendent, 1942.

66   BMICS, *Report for 1928*, p. 7.

67   BMICS, *Report for 1936*, p. 4.

68   BHF, *Report for 1939–1941*, inside front cover.

69   BSC, DM980 (30), Bristol Hospitals Commission, BHF evidence, appendix 7. Copies of the *Western Daily Press* and *Bristol Mirror*, 20 July 1939, 'Bristol Voluntary Hospitals, Contributory Scheme Inaugurated, Fund Which Will Embrace City and District'.

70   Royal Victoria Hospital, Annual Report for 1923 (Belfast, 1924), p. 16. See Donnacha Seán Lucey and George Campbell Gosling, 'Paying for health: comparative perspectives on patient payment and contributions for hospital provision in Ireland' in Donnacha Seán Lucey and Virginia Crossman (eds), *Healthcare in Ireland and Britain 1850–1970: Voluntary, Regional and Comparative Perspectives* (London: IHR, 2014), p. 87.

71   BMICS, *Report for 1929*, p. 8.

72   BSC, DM980 (5), Letter from Mr Dodd to Alderman Burgess, 14 May 1941; and Letter from Mr Dodd to Mr Iles of Torbay Hospitals Contributory Scheme, 3 April 1941.

73   BRO, Bristol Orthopaedic Hospital, *Reports for 1926–1927*; Winford Orthopaedic Hospital, *Reports for 1930–1940* and *1944–1947*.

74   BRO, Bristol Temporary Home and Lying-in Hospital, *Report for 1908*, p. 5 (original emphasis).

75   *Ibid., Reports for 1908–1939* (original emphasis).

76   Simon Gunn, *The Public Culture of the Victorian Middle Class: Ritual and Authority in the English Industrial City, 1840–1914* (Manchester: Manchester University Press, 2000), p. 182. See also Patrick Joyce, *The Rule of Freedom: Liberalism and the City in Britain* (London: Verso, 2003).

77   See Anne Rodrick, *Self-Help and Civic Culture: Citizenship in Victorian Birmingham* (Aldershot: Ashgate, 2004) for such an approach to the franchise and citizenship. On a similarly passive view of interwar citizenship, see Sian Nicholas, 'From John Bull to John Citizen: Images of National Identity and Citizenship on the Wartime BBC' in Richard Weight and Abigail Beach, *The Right to Belong: Citizenship and National Identity in Britain, 1930–1960* (London: I.B. Taurus, 1998), pp. 46–58.

78   See Glen O'Hara, 'The Complexities of "Consumerism": Choice, Collectivism and Participation within Britain's National Health Service,

c.1961–1979', *Social History of Medicine*, 26:2 (2013), 288–304; and Alex Mold, 'Patient Groups and the Construction of the Patient-Consumer in Britain: An Historical Overview', *Journal of Social Policy*, 39:4 (2010), 505–21.

79 Geoffrey Finlayson, 'A Moving Frontier: Voluntarism and the State in British Social Welfare, 1911–1949', *Twentieth Century British History*, 1:2 (1990), 194.

80 Tom Hulme, 'Civic Culture and Citizenship: The Nature of Urban Governance in Interwar Manchester and Chicago', unpublished PhD thesis, University of Leicester, 2013, p. 123.

81 Jim Cobley, 'Happy Birthday NHS', TSSA (Transport and Salaried Staffs' Association) Journal, August/September 2008, http://www.tssa.org.uk/article-269.php3?id_article=4349, accessed 9 September 2010; Cherry, 'Accountability', p. 230.

82 BMICS, *Report for 1928*, p. 7.

83 BMICS, *Report for 1936*, p. 6.

84 BMICS, *Report for 1937*, inside back cover.

85 Gorsky and Mohan, *Mutualism and Health Care*, pp. 65 and 108.

86 Barry M. Doyle, 'Power and Accountability in the Voluntary Hospitals of Middlesbrough 1900–48' in Peter Shapely and Anne Borsay (ed.), *Medicine, Charity and Mutual Aid: The Consumption of Health and Welfare, c.1550–1950* (Aldershot: Ashgate, 2006), p. 210.

87 Gorsky, Mohan and Willis, *Mutualism and Health Care*, p. 109.

88 William Beveridge, *Voluntary Action* (London: Allen & Unwin, 1948), p. 292.

89 *Ibid.*, p. 93.

90 Cherry, 'Accountability', pp. 230–1; Mohan and Gorsky, *Mutualism and Health Care*, p. 108; Doyle, 'Power and Accountability'.

91 BSC, DM980 (35), BHF, central contributory scheme memorandum, 1939. Different membership figures for 1938 of 250,000 for the Merseyside Hospitals Council rather than the Sheffield Hospitals Council and 700,000 compared to 600,000 for the Birmingham Hospitals Contributory Association appear in Gorsky and Mohan, *Mutualism and Health Care*, p. 44. Whichever of these figures are more accurate, they are significantly larger than those for Bristol.

92 BSC, Bristol Hospitals Commission, BHF evidence, appendix 22.

93 BHF, *Reports for 1939–1948*.

94 Gorsky and Mohan, *Mutualism and Health Care*, p. 72.

95 Tout, *Standard of Living*; Madge, 'Propensity to Save', p. 411.

96 Madge, 'Propensity to Save', p. 416.

97 Beier, *For Their Own Good*, p. 136. The term 'get free treatment' is used in the cited text.

98 Beveridge noted the 'double significance' in *Voluntary Action*, p. 116.

99 On the skill required for and pride taken in managing domestic resources, see for example Joanne Bourke, *Working-Class Cultures in Britain 1890–1960: Gender, Class and Ethnicity* (London: Routledge, 1994), pp. 62–7; Ellen Ross *Love and Toil: Motherhood in Outcast London, 1870–1918* (Oxford: Oxford University Press, 1993), pp. 40–55; Deirdre Beddoe, *Back to Home and Duty: Women between the Wars, 1918–1939* (London: Pandora, 1989), pp. 99–101.

100 W.J. Braithwaite quoted in Fraser, *Evolution*, p. 177.

101 For the most thorough discussion of the 1911 Act, see Gilbert Bentley, *The Evolution of National Insurance in Great Britain: The Origins of the Welfare State* (London: M. Joseph, 1966).

102 Hilaire Belloc, *The Servile State* (London: T.N. Foulis, 1912), pp. 164–5. Online version available at http://www.archive.org/details/servilestate-00belluoft, accessed 8 November 2015.

103 Cited in Pat Thane, *Foundations of the Welfare State*, 2nd edition (Harlow: Longman, 1996), p. 57.

104 Fraser, *Evolution*, p. 177.

105 Mark Abrams, *The Condition of the British People 1911–1945* (London: Victor Gollancz, 1946), pp. 84–5.

106 Fraser, *Evolution*, p. 177.

107 *Ibid.*, p. 212.

108 Steven Thompson, 'Varieties of Voluntarism in the South Wales Coalfield, c.1880–1914' in Colin Rochester, George Campbell Gosling, Alison Penn and Meta Zimmeck (eds.), *Understanding the Roots of Voluntary Action: Historical Perspectives on Current Social Policy* (Brighton: Sussex Academic Press, 2011), pp. 82–94.

109 Gareth Stedman Jones, *Outcast London: A Study in the Relationship between Classes in Victorian Society* (Oxford: Oxford University Press, 1971).

110 See R.J. Morris, 'Governance: Two Centuries of Urban Growth' in R.J. Morris and R.H. Trainor, *Urban Governance: Britain and Beyond since 1750* (Aldershot: Ashgate, 2000), p. 10.

111 See Nick Hayes and Barry M. Doyle, 'Eggs, Rags and Whist Drives: Popular Munificence and the Development of Provincial Medical Voluntarism between the Wars', *Historical Research*, 86:234 (2013), 625–61.

112 Tom Hulme, 'Civic Culture', p. 30.

113 Beck, *Almoner*, p. 61.

114 BRI, *Report for 1921*, p. 20.

115 See Anne Digby, *Making a Medical Living: Doctors and Patients in the English Market for Medicine, 1720–1911* (Cambridge: Cambridge University Press, 1994), p. 125.

116 Digby, *Evolution*, 245.

117 BRI Faculty Minutes, 16 November 1927, 15 June 1932.

118 *Ibid.*, 4 June 1928.

119 MRC, MSS.378/IMSW/A/15/13/4a: Institute of Almoners, Report on Replies to the Questionnaire, 'The Functions of an Almoner', 1947.

120 MRC, MSS.378/IMSW/A/15/13/4a: Institute of Almoners, Functions Committee.

121 MRC, MSS.378/IMSW/A/16/4/1: Institute of Almoners, 'Important Statement', 21 February 1952. Original emphasis.

122 MRC, MSS.378/IMSW/A/16/4/2: Institute of Almoners, 'Report of the Emergency Professional Meeting Held on 19th April 1952'.

123 MRC, MSS.378/IMSW/A/16/4/8: Telegram from Ministry of Health to the Institute of Almoners, 'proposed Charges for Hospital Appliances, etc.', 21 May 1952.

124 Cited in Charles Webster, *The National Health Service: A Political History*, 2nd revised edition (Oxford: Oxford University Press, 2002), p. 24.

125 Clement Attlee, 'The New Social Services and the Citizen', 4 July 1948, *BBC Archive: Birth of the National Health Service*, http://www.bbc.co.uk/archive/nhs/5147.shtml, accessed 25 April 2016.

Conclusion

Between his time working in the Clyde shipyards and writing a quintet of novels on the life of Robert Burns, James Barke wrote a little-remembered saga of Glasgow life called *Major Operation*. In this 1930s novel, two characters are brought together on the wards of the Eastern Infirmary (presumably the thinly veiled Western Infirmary, one of the city's three large general voluntary hospitals and the only one without private wards). Jock MacKelvie is an unemployed leader, rushed to the hospital after a fall at a political rally. George Anderson is an international coal trader on the verge of bankruptcy as a victim of global economic turbulence. When George suffers abdominal pain and calls out the doctor in the night, he has to 'confess' that he cannot afford a nursing home, but must instead 'trust himself to the tender mercies of a public charitable institution.'[1]

George's expectation that 'there would be a lot of scandal' once 'his friends got to know he was lying in the Eastern beside the riff-raff of the Second City' was matched by the attitude of the nurse taking his details when admitted.[2] When he gave an address in a well-heeled part of town, 'She turned and gave him a sour look. A snob: pride and poverty.'[3] Once on Ward 101, the other patients thought him a 'toff' and a 'swell guy', but found him 'quite a decent fellow'.[4] Meanwhile, the surgeon was 'interested' in George, who was 'so obviously middle class. And he guessed he must have been pretty low' for his doctor to have sent him there. As a poor patient of middle-class character, the surgeon knew 'Anderson would get the same skill – if not the same nursing – for nothing.' He explained the medical details 'to the students who, recognising Anderson as one of their own class, felt slightly uncomfortable.'[5]

The overarching narrative of the book is of a democratic transformation, with the classes brought together and a radical change in middle-
class political outlook the result. George realises he 'had always been a
snob, even if a humane one. He had always instinctively recognised the
gulf that lay beneath the classes. Never under any circumstances had he
made any attempt to bridge the gulf himself or allow it to be bridged
from the other side.'[6] The hospital serves as a democratic space within
which this can happen – but only because financial difficulties remove
him from his natural class. The novel is essentially utopian, in that it has
to contrive an interruption in the established order to provide the
premise on which the events unfold. That established order is the class
differentiation we have seen to be a defining characteristic of the
pre-NHS hospitals. Despite the changes taking place in the early twentieth century, the admission of patients of all classes alongside each
other did not become the norm, nor were the hospitals taken over by
work geared towards the accommodation or treatment of those who
could pay a commercial rate, as in America. The hospital did not become
a site for generating profit. Yet payment did find a place, even as the
hospital remained essentially a philanthropic institution.

The idea that the working classes should pay in to the system, the
various schemes that facilitated this in the community and the almoner
who policed it in the hospital, as well as the idea of opening up the
hospital to middle-class patients, were all inventions of the nineteenth
century. Yet it was not until the interwar years that any of them became
the norm, or even commonplace. In both principle and practice, the
change brought about was more complex than a simple switch from
medical charity to private healthcare – a reformulation rather than a
rejection of philanthropy.

Philanthropy reformulated

The voluntary hospitals underwent a great many changes during the
interwar years. Those in the medical technology they employed were
matched by changing dynamics in relations with the local and national
state, while new styles of fundraising fostered a more democratic relationship with the local community.[7] As far the terms of access to the
hospitals were concerned, the change can be understood essentially as
the adoption of *economic reciprocalism*. Medical need and inability to

receive the necessary treatment beyond the walls of the hospital had never been the only criteria for admission, but the early twentieth century saw a change in what the others were. In the late nineteenth century they had been focused on socio-behavioural expectations which demonstrated deservingness. The early twentieth century saw them gradually give way to financial contribution. To be a contributor not only proved that one was not a *free-rider*, it also denoted self-sufficiency and sound management of household finances. In short, it was the mark of a good citizen. A universal right to healthcare was beyond the reach of this notion of citizenship, even as medical provision was made to ever-greater numbers drawn from new sections of the community. Indeed, it is responsibilities rather than rights that appear to have been more prominent.

This delicate balance was policed by the almoner, and the foundation and expansion of the almoner profession was inextricably bound up with the administration of payment schemes. She arrived in the hospital to identify those who could afford to pay the cost of their treatment and assess those who might be able to make a lesser contribution. Her qualification for doing so (as well as two years of university study and a series of hospital placements) was her understanding of the patient not simply as research material or as a medical consumer, but within their wider social circumstances. She both enforced payment and acted to protect the patient against its unfair implementation. When the profession's national body changed its name from the Institute of Almoners to the Institute of Medical Social Workers in 1964 it was in fact a long-overdue recognition of the nature of their work, just as when the NHS removed their financial function it did not leave them struggling to find a new purpose. By 1948 the almoners were ready to make the case that any business related to patient payments was a distraction from their real work in the hospital, a view the medical profession had long held. Financial and social work were dual strands, each deeply rooted. Both were indicative elements of the hospitals as charities, but only the latter was equally as applicable to working in the NHS. The social function of the hospital both provided the cover for the compassionate introduction of a financial dimension to the patient contract and ensured the social worker's continued usefulness after its abolition.

This continued social function is inseparable from a commitment to prioritise the treatment of the sick poor. Exactly what was meant by the *sick poor*, however, was not static. The broadening of the patient base, although more limited than might have been expected, was sufficient to prompt a redefinition. While some of those admitted to the private wards fell well beyond any definition of *poor*, it was promoted by the champions of private practice as a philanthropic function of the hospital to leave nobody (even the wealthy) without the latest, most technologically equipped medical care at times of need. More widely and more convincingly it was understood that this coincided with demographic and economic changes that meant many of those previously able to pay for home visits from their doctor now needed to turn to the hospital. As the costs of medical care rose along with many others, the *new poor* of the lower middle classes, when taken sick, could now be thought of as the *new sick poor*. Those financially incapable of securing medical treatment, the meaning of the term *sick poor* as it was commonly used in the early twentieth century, was a genuinely growing category. At a time of medical, technological and socio-economic change, medical charity changed too.

Philanthropy maintained

Yet the voluntary hospitals neither adopted a commercial emphasis nor evolved a universal service, even as the hospital was opened up to patients of all classes. The pursuit of those new patients most able to benefit the hospitals financially was timid and consequently, as the evidence presented here has shown, private hospital services before the NHS never broke out from being marginal within the institution, largely restricted to the south of England and strikingly limited overall. With provision for middle-class patients no more than 3 or 4 per cent of pre-NHS hospital beds, the main work of Britain's hospitals continued until 1948 to be the treatment of the sick poor. And perhaps we should not be surprised to find the medical profession keen on maintaining this focus in their hospital work. Lucrative opportunities for private practice came from holding an honorary position at a major hospital, treating the full range of acute cases across the local population.[8] This meant a hard-nosed business interest in keeping access as open as possible, but it also meant trading off the philanthropic respectability garnered for the medical profession. Yet the scepticism and sometimes, as in Bristol, outright opposition of house committees to the admission of private patients is in stark contrast to the US case where Charles Rosenberg and Paul Starr have both identified the surgical staffs as driving the change, bringing their private patients to the hospital where it was more efficient and profitable to treat them.[9] There is little reason to think the same logic would not apply across the Atlantic. Yet the separation of their honorary, gratuitous hospital work from their private practice beyond was only occasionally broken. This was likely an important factor in the remarkably limited growth of the only truly commercial element of inpatient hospital provision.

Ensuring a universal service was not developed ahead of the NHS were a set of practical arrangements embodying the principle of *class differentiation*. These ensured that, even when the medical care of all classes was brought within the hospital, their separation and the distinction between the treatment of each was not abandoned. It was simply brought, to a limited extent, in-house. The clamour and sociability of the dormitory-style ordinary ward remained the setting for working-class hospital stays, while the middle-class experience of home treatment was, whenever possible, recreated as faithfully in the hospital as it was in the nursing home. Working-class patients continued to receive subsidised care, even when they made some financial contribution. Middle-class patients still had to negotiate a fee, but were safe in the knowledge that they would not be used as teaching material. The experiences of each, as well as their expectations and those placed upon them, were not the same and did not become so.

However, we should not regard these separations and distinctions as safeguards, limiting the move away from the traditional work and character of the voluntary hospital. In fact, the new practices associated with payment served to reinforce those traditions as they daily acted out the old class distinctions on which the social relationships of philanthropy are based. These new developments reasserting old principles served to mediate the adoption of universalism. As such, the pre-NHS practice of patient payments was rather different from today's medical consumerism, with an increasing tendency to view health as a 'commodity' and patients as 'consumers'.[10] Although this view is far from uncontested, debates around medical consumerism have formed an unhelpfully anachronistic backdrop to historical study in recent decades. The pre-NHS citizen patient was distinctly different, with the civic duty to contribute financially itself mediated by class. For those categorised as middle-class (a category assumed to be unproblematically aligned with higher income) there was an absolute obligation to pay. On the part of the roughly four-fifths of the population below the income limits, the most important thing was willingness to pay if possible, as demonstrated either by submission to the almoner's assessment or by membership of a contributory scheme. For the two preceding centuries, this same act of submission, demonstrating deservingness of medical charity, was played out in requesting a subscriber's ticket.[11] That role was now brought on-site and taken on by the almoner. Although this increasingly became a financial rather than behavioural code, adherence was still put on display to receive free treatment at the hospital. While demonstrable deference or even gratitude were deemed proper, the new patient contract ultimately required only acquiescence. Philanthropy still mediated the terms on which admission was gained.

This was just one way in which the dual role of patient and recipient of medical charity continued to be a passive one throughout the early twentieth century. What might initially appear commercial or mutual mechanisms for seizing control in the name of the patient, were in fact medically and socially governed as before. Hospital contributory schemes operated as an alternative to the almoner's assessment, opting out of the means-test to determine the terms of admission, but not securing admission itself. Meanwhile, there was no choice involved in the middle-class patient's more luxurious parallel accommodation. It was only the working-class patient with enough savings to pay for a private ward who could break free of the social hierarchies by which the hospital was bound. Overwhelming, they were reinforced rather than escaped. Payment in the voluntary hospitals was not the adoption of a consumer model of healthcare, but a bulwark against the development of the social democratic principle of patients as citizens with a right to treatment.

Notes

1 James Barke, *Major Operation: The Saga of a Scottish City* (London: Collins, 1955 [1936]), p. 145.
2 *Ibid.*, p. 158.
3 *Ibid.*, p. 146.
4 *Ibid.*, p. 160.

5 *Ibid.*, pp. 185–6.

6 *Ibid.*, p. 193.

7 Martin Gorsky, 'The Political Economy of Health Care in the Nineteenth and Twentieth Centuries' in Mark Jackson (ed.), *The Oxford Handbook of the History of Medicine* (Oxford: Oxford University Press, 2011), p. 435; Nick Hayes and Barry M. Doyle, 'Eggs, Rags and Whist Drives: Popular Munificence and the Development of Provincial Medical Voluntarism between the Wars', *Historical Research*, 86:234 (2013), 712–40.

8 See Anne Digby, *Making a Medical Living: Doctors and Patients in the English Market for Medicine, 1720–1911* (Cambridge: Cambridge University Press, 1994), pp. 125 and 135.

9 Charles Rosenberg, *The Care of Strangers: The Rise of America's Hospital System* (New York: Johns Hopkins University Press, 1987), pp. 237–61; Paul Starr, *The Social Transformation of American Medicine* (New York: Basic Books, 1982), p. 157. Rosenberg, *Care of Strangers*, pp. 237–61.

10 Saras Henderson and Alan Petersen, 'Introduction: Consumerism in Health Care' in Saras Henderson and Alan Petersen (eds), *Consuming Health: The Commodification of Health Care* (London: Routledge, 2002), p. 1.

11 Mary Fissell, *Patients, Power, and the Poor in Eighteenth-Century Bristol* (Cambridge: Cambridge University Press, 1991), p. 7.

Select bibliography

Primary sources

Unpublished

Bristol Record Office
29491, Records of the Bristol Hospitals Fund.
35893, Records of the Bristol Royal Infirmary.
40530, Records of the Bristol General Hospital.
37424, Records of the Bristol Royal Hospital for Sick Children and Women.

Bristol Reference Library
Bristol Council Minutes.
Bristol Health Committee Minute Book.
Bristol Medical Officer of Health Reports.

University of Bristol Special Collections
DM980, Records of the Bristol and District Divisional Hospitals Council and
　　Bristol Hospitals Fund.

London Metropolitan Archives
A/KE, Records of the King Edward's Hospital Fund for London.

Modern Records Centre, University of Warwick
MSS.378/IMSW, Records of the Institute of Medical Social Workers,
　　1895–1971.
Alan Cohen, 'Social Workers Speak Out' interviews (1980–81), https://www2
　　.warwick.ac.uk/services/library/mrc/explorefurther/speakingarchives/
　　socialwork/, accessed 25 April 2016.

The National Archive
MH 66/1068, 'County Borough of Bristol' Allan C Parsons (Ministry of
　　Health, 1932).

Published

Anon., *The Hospital Almoner: A Brief Study of Hospital Social Service in Great Britain* (London: Hospital Almoners Association, 1935).

Anon., *The Hospitals Year-Books* (London: Central Bureau of Hospital Information, 1933–47).

Burdett, Henry, *Pay Hospitals and Paying Wards throughout the World: Facts in Support of a Re-Arrangement of the English System of Medical Relief* (London: J.&A. Churchill, 1879).

Hospital Commission, *First General Report, 1933–34* (Dublin, 1936).

Ministry of Health

Carling, Ernest Rock and T.S. McIntosh, *Hospital Survey: The Hospital Services of the NorthWestern Area* (London, 1945).

Consultative Council on Medical and Allied Services, *Interim Report on the Future Provision of Medical and Allied Services* (London, 1920).

Cope, V. Zachary, W.J. Gill, Arthur Griffiths and G.C. Kelly, *Hospital Survey: The Hospital Services of the South-Western Area* (London, 1945).

Eason, Herbert, R. Veitch Clark and W.H. Harper, *Hospital Survey: The Hospital Services of the Yorkshire Area* (London, 1945).

Gray, A.M.H. and A. Topping, *Hospital Survey: The Hospital Services of London and the Surrounding Area* (London, 1945).

Jones, A. Trevor, J.A. Nixon and R.M.F. Picken, *Hospital Survey: The Hospital Services of South Wales and Monmouthshire* (Welsh Board of Health, 1945).

Savage, Willam G., Claude Frankau and Basil Gibson, *Hospital Survey: The Hospital Services of the Eastern Area* (London, 1945).

Nuffield Provincial Hospitals Trust, *The Hospital Surveys: The Domesday Book of Hospital Services* (Oxford: Oxford University Press, 1946).

Political and Economic Planning, *Report on the British Health Services* (London: PEP, 1937).

Strachey, Ray, *Careers and Openings for Women: A Survey of Women's Employment and a Guide for Those Seeking Work* (London: Faber and Faber, 1935).

Online

Halas, John and Joy Batchelor, *Your Very Good Health* (Central Office of Information, 1948), http://film.wellcome.ac.uk:15151/mediaplayer.html?0055-0000-4225-0115-0-0000-0000-0, accessed 25 April 2016.

Rivett, Geoffrey, *The Development of the London Hospital System, 1823–1982* (London: King's Fund, 1982), http://www.nhshistory.net/Londonshospitals.htm, accessed 25 April 2016.

Secondary works

Abel-Smith, Brian, *The Hospitals 1800–1948* (London: Heinemann, 1964).

Abrams, Mark, *The Conditions of the British People, 1911–1945* (London: Victor Gollancz, 1946).

Beck, I.F., *The Almoner: A Brief Account of Medical Social Service in Great Britain* (London: Council of the Institute of Almoners, 1948).

Beier, Lucinda McCray, *For Their Own Good: The Transformation of English Working-Class Health Culture, 1880–1970* (Columbus: Ohio State University Press, 2008).

Beveridge, William, *Voluntary Action* (London: Allen & Unwin, 1948).

Bickerton, Thomas H., *A Medical History of Liverpool from the Earliest Days to the Year 1920* (London: J. Murray, 1936).

Bourke, Joanne, *Working-Class Cultures in Britain 1890–1960: Gender, Class and Ethnicity* (London: Routledge, 1994).

Bridgen, Paul, 'Voluntary Failure, the Middle Classes, and the Nationalisation of the British Voluntary Hospitals, 1900–1946' in Bernard Harris and Paul Bridgen (eds), *Charity and Mutual Aid in Europe and North America since 1800* (London: Routledge, 2007), pp. 212–34.

Bruce Perry, C., *Voluntary Medical Institutions* (Bristol: Bristol Branch of the Historical Association, 1984).

Cherry, Steven, 'Beyond National Health Insurance. The Voluntary Hospitals and Hospital Contributory Schemes: A Regional Study', *Social History of Medicine*, 5:3 (1992), 455–82.

Cherry, Steven, 'Accountability, Entitlement, and Control Issues and Voluntary Hospital Funding c1860–1939', *Social History of Medicine*, 9:2 (1996), 215–33.

Cherry, Steven, *Medical Services and the Hospital in Britain, 1860–1939* (Cambridge: Cambridge University Press, 1996).

Cherry, Steven, 'Before the National Health Service: Financing the Voluntary Hospitals, 1900–1939', *Economic History Review*, 50:2 (1997), 305–26.

Cherry, Steven, 'Hospital Saturday, Workplace Collections and Issues in Late Nineteenth-Century Hospital Funding', *Medical History*, 44:4 (2000), 461–88.

Clarke, Charles, *Bristol Royal Infirmary: A Personal Study Written to Commemorate the First 250 Years, 1735–1985* (Bristol: Portishead Press, 1985).

Cullen, Lynsey, 'The First Lady Almoner: The Appointment, Position, and Findings of Miss Mary Stewart at the Royal Free Hospital, 1895–99', *Journal of the History of Medicine and Allied Sciences*, 68:4 (2013), 551–82.

Daunton, Martin, 'Payment and Participation: Welfare and State-Formation in Britain, 1990–1951', *Past and Present*, 150 (1990), 188–91.

DiGaetano, Alan, 'The Birth of Modern Urban Governance: A Comparison of Political Modernization in Boston, Massachusetts, and Bristol, England, 1800–1870', *Journal of Urban History*, 35:2 (2009), 259–87.

Digby, Anne, *Making a Medical Living: Doctors and Patients in the English Market for Medicine, 1720–1911* (Cambridge: Cambridge University Press, 1994).

Digby, Anne, *The Evolution of British General Practice, 1850–1948* (Oxford: Oxford University Press, 1999).

Digby, Anne and Nick Bosanquet, 'Doctors and Patients in an Era of National Health Insurance and Private Practice, 1913–1938', *Economic History Review*, 41:1 (1988), 74–95.

Dow, D.A., M.M. Leitch and A.F. MacLean, *From Almoner to Social Worker: Social Work at Glasgow Royal Infirmary, 1932–1982* (Glasgow: Glasgow Royal Infirmary, 1982).

Doyle, Barry M., *A History of Hospitals in Middlesbrough* (Middlesbrough: South Tees NHS Hospitals Trust, 2003).

Doyle, Barry M., 'Power and Accountability in the Voluntary Hospitals of Middlesborough 1900–48' in Peter Shapely and Anne Borsay (ed.), *Medicine, Charity and Mutual Aid: The Consumption of Health and Welfare, c.1550–1950* (Aldershot: Ashgate, 2006), pp. 207–24.

Doyle, Barry M., 'Competition and Cooperation in Hospital Provision in Middlesbrough, 1918–1948', *Medical History*, 51:3 (2007), 337–56.

Doyle, Barry M., 'Labour and Hospitals in Three Yorkshire Towns: Middlesbrough, Leeds, Sheffield, 1919–1938', *Social History of Medicine*, 23:2 (2010), 374–92.

Doyle, Barry M., *The Politics of Hospital Provision in Early 20th-Century Britain* (London: Pickering and Chatto, 2014).

Doyle, Barry M., 'Healthcare before Welfare States: Hospitals in Early Twentieth Century England and France', *Canadian Bulletin of Medical History*, 33:1 (2016), 174–204.

Dresser, Madge, 'People's Housing in Bristol, 1870–1939' in Ian Bild (ed.), *Bristol's Other History* (Bristol: Bristol Broadsides, 1983), pp. 129–60.

Eversley, John, 'The History of NHS Charges', *Contemporary British History*, 15:2 (2001), 53–75.

Finlayson, Geoffrey, 'A Moving Frontier: Voluntarism and the State in British Social Welfare, 1911–1949', *Twentieth Century British History*, 1:2 (1990), 183–206.

Finlayson, Geoffrey, *Citizen, State, and Social Welfare in Britain 1830–1990* (Oxford: Oxford University Press, 1994).

Fissell, Mary, *Patients, Power, and the Poor in Eighteenth-Century Bristol* (Cambridge: Cambridge University Press, 1991).

Fissell, Mary, 'Charity Universal? Institutions and Moral Reform in Eighteenth-Century Bristol' in Lee Davison, Tim Hitchcock, Tim Keirn and Robert Shoemaker (eds), *Still The Grumbling Hive: The Response to Social and Economic Problems in England, 1689–1750* (Stroud: St Martin's Press, 1992), pp. 121–64.

Fissell, Mary, 'The Disappearance of the Patient Narrative and the Invention of Hospital Medicine' in Roger French and Andrew Wear (eds), *British Medicine in an Age of Reform* (London: Routledge, 2002), pp. 92–109.

Foucade, Marion, and Kieran Healey, 'Moral Views of Market Society', *Annual Review of Sociology*, 33 (2007), 285–311.

Fox, Daniel M., *Health Policies, Health Politics: The British and American Experience, 1911–1965* (Princeton: Princeton University Press, 1986).

Gorsky, Martin, *Patterns of Philanthropy: Charity and Society in Nineteenth-Century Bristol* (Woodbridge: Boydell & Brewer Ltd, 1999).

Gorsky, Martin, ' "For the Treatment of Sick Persons of All Classes": The Transformation of Bristol's Hospital Services, 1918–1939' in Peter Wardley (ed.), *Bristol Historical Resource*, CD-ROM (Bristol: University of the West of England, 2001).

Gorsky, Martin, ' "Threshold of a New Era": The Development of an Integrated Hospital System in Northeast Scotland, 1900–1939', *Social History of Medicine*, 17:2 (2004), 247–67.

Gorsky, Martin, 'The Gloucestershire Extension of Medical Services Scheme: An Experiment in the Integration of Health Services in Britain before the NHS', *Medical History*, 50:4 (2006), 491–512.

Gorsky, Martin, 'The Political Economy of Health Care in the Nineteenth and Twentieth Centuries' in Mark Jackson (ed.), *The Oxford Handbook of the History of Medicine* (Oxford: Oxford University Press, 2011), pp. 429–49.

Gorsky, Martin, John Mohan and Martin Powell, 'British Voluntary Hospitals 1871–1939: The Geography of Provision and Utilization', *Journal of Historical Geography*, 25:4 (1999), 463–82.

Gorsky, Martin, John Mohan and Martin Powell, 'The Financial Health of Voluntary Hospitals in Interwar Britain', *Economic History Review*, 55:3 (2002), 533–57.

Gorsky, Martin, Martin Powell and John Mohan, 'British Voluntary Hospitals and the Public Sphere: Contribution and Participation before the National Health Service' in Steve Sturdy (ed.), *Medicine, Health and the Public Sphere in Britain 1600–2000* (London: Routledge, 2002), pp. 123–44.

Gorsky, Martin, John Mohan and Tim Willis, 'From Hospital Contributory Schemes to Health Cash Plans: The Mutual Ideal in British Health Care after 1948', *Journal of Social Policy*, 34:3 (2005), 447–67.

Gorsky, Martin, John Mohan and Tim Willis, 'Hospital Contributory Schemes and the NHS Debates 1937–46: The Rejection of Social Insurance in the British Welfare State?', *Twentieth Century British History*, 16:2 (2005), 170–92.

Gorsky, Martin, John Mohan with Tim Willis, *Mutualism and Health Care: British Hospital Contributory Schemes in the Twentieth Century* (Manchester: Manchester University Press, 2006).

Gosling, George Campbell, 'The Patient Contract in Bristol's Voluntary Hospitals, c.1918–1929', *University of Sussex Journal of Contemporary History*, 11 (2007), 1–16.

Gosling, George Campbell, ' "Open the Other Eye": Payment, Civic Duty and Hospital Contributory Schemes in Bristol, c.1927–1948', *Medical History*, 54:4 (2010), 475–494.

Gosling, George Campbell, 'Charity and Change in the Mixed Economy of Healthcare in Bristol, 1918–1948', unpublished PhD thesis, Oxford Brookes University, 2011.

Gosling, George Campbell, 'The Birth of the Pregnant Patient-Consumer? Payment, Paternalism and Maternity Hospitals in Early Twentieth-Century England' in Jennifer Evans and Ciara Meehan (eds), *Perceptions of Pregnancy from the Seventeenth to Twentieth Century* (London: Palgrave Macmillan, 2016).

Granovetter, Mark, 'Economic Action and Social Structure: The Problem of Embeddedness', *American Journal of Sociology*, 91:3 (1985), 481–510.

Granshaw, Lindsay, ' "Fame and Fortune by Means of Bricks and Mortar": The Medical Profession and Specialist Hospitals in Britain, 1800–1948' in Lindsay Granshaw and Roy Porter (eds), *The Hospital in History* (London: Routledge, 1989), pp. 199–220.

Hamilton, David, 'The Highlands and Islands Medical Service' in Gordon McLachlan (ed.), *Improving the Common Weal: Aspects of Scottish Health Services 1900–1984* (Edinburgh: Edinburgh University Press, 1987), pp. 483–90.

Harvey, Philip and Jon Press, 'Industrial Change and the Economic Life of Bristol since 1800' in Charles Harvey and Jon Press (eds), *Studies in the Business History of Bristol* (Bristol: Bristol Academic Press, 1988), pp. 1–32.

Hayes, Nick, 'Did We Really Want a National Health Service? Hospitals, Patients and Public Opinions before 1948', *English Historical Review*, 128:526 (2012), 625–61.

Hayes, Nick, ' "Our Hospitals"? Voluntary Provision, Community and Civic Consciousness in Nottingham Before the NHS', *Midland History*, 37:1 (2012), 84–105.

Hayes, Nick and Barry M. Doyle, 'Eggs, Rags and Whist Drives: Popular Munificence and the Development of Provincial Medical Voluntarism between the Wars', *Historical Research*, 86:234 (2013), 712–40.

Hazlehurst, John, 'Health Inequalities in Bristol 1918–1939' in Wardley (ed.), *Bristol Historical Resource*, CD-ROM (Bristol: University of the West of England, 2001).

Hickman, Clare, *Therapeutic Landscapes: A History of English Hospital Gardens since 1800* (Manchester: Manchester University Press, 2013).

Hodgkinson, Ruth, *The Origins of the National Health Service: The Medical Services of the New Poor Law, 1834–1871* (London: Wellcome Historical Medical Library, 1967).

Jones, Colin, 'Some Recent Trends in the History of Charity', in Martin Daunton (ed.), *Charity, Self-Interest and Welfare in the English Past* (London: UCL Press, 1996), pp. 51–63.

Kidd, Alan, 'Philanthropy and the "Social History Paradigm"', *Social History*, 2:2 (1996), 180–92.

Large, David, *The Municipal Government of Bristol, 1851–1901* (Bristol: Bristol Record Society, 1999).

Levene, Alysa, 'Between Less Eligibility and the NHS: The Changing Place of Poor Law Hospitals in England and Wales, 1929–39', *Twentieth Century British History*, 20:3 (1997), 322–45.

Levene, Alysa, Martin Powell and John Stewart, 'Patterns of Municipal Health Expenditure in Interwar England and Wales', *Bulletin of the History of Medicine*, 78:3 (2004), 635–66.

Levene, Alysa, Martin Powell, John Stewart and Becky Taylor, *From Cradle to Grave: Municipal Provision in Interwar England and Wales* (Bern: Peter Lang, 2011).

Lewis, Richard, Robina Nixon and Barry M. Doyle, *Health Services in Middlesbrough: North Ormesby Hospital 1900–1948* (Middlesbrough: Centre for Local Historical Research, University of Teesside, 1999).

Lucey, Donnacha Seán and George Campbell Gosling, 'Paying for Health: Comparative Perspectives on Patient Payment and Contributions for Hospital Provision in Ireland' in Donnacha Seán Lucey and Virginia Crossman (eds), *Healthcare in Ireland and Britain from 1850: Voluntary, Regional and Comparative Perspectives* (London: Institute of Historical Research, 2015), pp. 81–100.

Madge, Charles, 'The Propensity to Save in Blackburn and Bristol', *Economic Journal*, 50:200 (1940), 410–48.

Manchée, Dorothy, *Whatever Does the Almoner Do?* (London: Bailliere, Tindall and Cox., 1946).

Marks, Lara, ' "They're magicians". Midwives, Doctors and Hospitals: Women's Experience of Childbirth in East London and Woolwich in the Interwar Years', *Oral History*, 23 (1995), 46–53.

Marks, Lara, *Metropolitan Maternity: Maternal and Infant Welfare Service in Early Twentieth Century London* (Amsterdam: Rodopi, 1996).

Marland, Hilary, *Medicine and Society in Wakefield and Huddersfield, 1780–1870* (Cambridge: Cambridge University Press, 1987).

Marland, Hilary, 'Lay and Medical Conceptions of Medical Charity during the Nineteenth Century' in Jonathan Barry and Colin Jones (eds), *Medicine and Charity before the Welfare State* (London: Routledge, 1991), pp. 149–71.

Marland, Hilary, 'The Changing Role of the Hospital, 1800–1900' in Deborah Brunton (ed.), *Medicine Transformed: Health, Disease and Society in Europe 1800–1930* (Manchester: Manchester University Press, 2004), pp. 31–60.

Marmion, V.J., *The Bristol Eye Hospital: A Monograph* (Bristol, 1987).

Martin, Moira, 'Managing the Poor: The Administration of Poor Relief in Bristol in the Nineteenth and Twentieth Centuries' in Madge Dresser and Philip Ollerenshaw (eds), *The Making of Modern Bristol* (Bristol: Redcliffe Press, 1996), pp. 156–83.

McIntosh, Tania, *A Social History of Maternity and Childbirth: Key Themes in Maternity Care* (London: Routledge, 2012).

Meller, Helen, *Leisure and the Changing City, 1870–1914* (London: Routledge and Kegan Paul, 1976).

Moberly Bell, Enid, *The Story of Hospital Almoners: The Birth of a Profession* (London: Faber & Faber, 1961).

Mohan, John, *Planning, Markets and Hospitals* (London: Routledge, 2002).

Mohan, John and Martin Gorsky, *Don't Look Back? Voluntary and Charitable Finance of Hospital in Britain, Past and Present* (London: Office of Health Economics & Association of Chartered Certified Accountants, 2001).

Nottingham, Chris and Rona Dougall, 'A Close and Practical Association with the Medical Profession: Scottish Medical Social Workers and the Social Medicine, 1940–1975', *Medical History*, 51:3 (2007), 309–36.

Nuttall, Alison, 'Taking "Advantage of the Facilities and Comforts … Offered": Women's Choice of Hospital Delivery in Interwar Edinburgh' in Janet Greenlees and Linda Bryder (eds), *Western Maternity 1880–1990* (London: Pickering & Chatto, 2013), pp. 65–80.

Ollerenshaw, Philip and Peter Wardley, 'Economic Growth and the Business Community in Bristol since 1840' in Madge Dresser and Philip Ollerenshaw (eds), *The Making of Modern Bristol* (Bristol: Redcliffe Press, 1996), pp. 124–55.

Owen, David, *English Philanthropy 1660–1960* (Cambridge, MA: Harvard University Press, 1966).

Pater, John, *The Making of the National Health Service* (London: King's Fund, 1981).

Peretz, Elizabeth, 'Maternal and Child Welfare in England and Wales between the Wars: A Comparative Regional Study', unpublished PhD thesis, Middlesex University, 1992.

Pickstone, John, *Medicine and Industrial Society: A History of Hospital Development in Manchester and Its Region* (Manchester: Manchester University Press, 1985).

Pinker, Robert, *English Hospital Statistics 1861–1938* (London: Heinemann, 1966).

Porter, Roy, 'The Gift Relation: Philanthropy and Provincial Hospitals in Eighteenth-Century England' in Lindsay Granshaw and Roy Porter (eds), *The Hospital in History* (London: Routledge, 1989), pp. 149–78.

Powell, Martin, 'An Expanding Service: Municipal Acute Medicine in the 1930s', *Twentieth Century British History*, 8:3 (1997), 334–57.

Powell, Martin, 'Coasts and Coalfields: The Geographical Distribution of Doctors in England and Wales in the 1930s', *Social History of Medicine*, 18:2 (2005), 245–63.

Prochaska, F., *Philanthropy and the Hospitals of London: The King's Fund, 1897–1990* (Oxford: Clarendon Press, 1992).

Prochaska, F., 'Burdett, Sir Henry Charles (1847–1920)', *Oxford Dictionary of National Biography*, Oxford: Oxford University Press, 2004, http://0-www.oxforddnb.com.pugwash.lib.warwick.ac.uk/view/article/38827, accessed 25 April 2016.

Reinarz, Jonathan, 'Charitable Bodies: The Funding of Birmingham's Voluntary Hospitals in the Nineteenth Century' in Martin Gorsky and Sally Sheard (eds), *Financing Medicine: The British Experience since 1750* (London: Routledge, 2006), pp. 40–58.

Reinarz, Jonathan, 'Investigating the "Deserving" Poor: Charity, Discipline and Voluntary Hospitals in Nineteenth-Century Birmingham' in Peter Shapely and Anne Borsay (ed.), *Medicine, Charity and Mutual Aid: The Consumption of Health and Welfare, c.1550–1950* (Aldershot: Ashgate, 2006), pp. 111–34.

Reinarz, Jonathan, *Health Care in Birmingham: The Birmingham Teaching Hospitals, 1779–1939* (Woodbridge: Boydell Press, 2014).

Risse, Guenter, *Mending Bodies, Saving Souls: A History of Hospitals* (Oxford: Oxford University Press, 1999).

Rivett, Geoffrey, *From Cradle to Grave: Fifty Years of the NHS* (London: King's Fund, 1997).

Rosenberg, Charles, *The Care of Strangers: The Rise of America's Hospital System* (New York: Johns Hopkins University Press, 1987).

Rosner, David, *A Once Charitable Enterprise: Hospitals and Health Care in Brooklyn and New York, 1885–1915* (Cambridge: Cambridge University Press, 1982).

Saunders, Charles, *The Bristol Eye Hospital* (Bristol: United Bristol Hospitals, 1960).

Saunders, Charles, *The Bristol Royal Hospital for Sick Children* (Bristol: United Bristol Hospitals, 1961).

Saunders, Charles, *The United Bristol Hospitals* (Bristol: United Bristol Hospitals, 1965).

Simmons, Angela, *A Profession and Its Roots: The Lady Almoners* (Michelangelo Press, 2005), https://www.kcl.ac.uk/sspp/policy-institute/scwru/swhn/publications/Simmons-A-Profession-and-Its-Roots-The-Lady-Almoners.pdf, accessed 25 April 2016.

Smith, Timothy B., *Creating the Welfare State in France, 1880–1940* (Montreal: McGill-Queen's University Press, 2003).

Starr, Paul, *The Social Transformation of American Medicine* (New York: Basic Books, 1982).

Stewart, John, '"For a Healthy London": The Socialist Medical Association and the London County Council in the 1930s', *Medical History*, 42:4 (1997), 417–36.

Stewart, John, *The Battle for Health': A Political History of the Socialist Medical Association, 1930–51* (Aldershot: Ashgate, 1999).

Stewart, John, 'Ideology and Process in the Creation of the British National Health Service', *Journal of Policy History*, 14:1 (2002), 113–34.

Stewart, John, '"The Finest Municipal Hospital Service in the World"?: Contemporary Perceptions of the London County Council's Hospital Provision, 1929–1939', *Urban History*, 32:2 (2005), 327–44.

Stewart, John, 'The Mixed Economy of Welfare in Historical Context' in Martin Powell (ed.), *Understanding the Mixed Economy of Welfare* (Bristol: Policy Press, 2007), pp. 23–40.

Thompson, Steven, 'A Proletarian Public Sphere: Working-Class Provision of Medical Services and Care in South Wales, c.1900–1948' in Anne Borsay (ed.), *Medicine in Wales c.1800–2000: Public Service or Private Commodity?* (Cardiff: University of Wales Press, 2003), pp. 86–107.

Thompson, Steven, 'Varieties of Voluntarism in the South Wales Coalfield, c.1880–1914' in Colin Rochester, George Campbell Gosling, Alison Penn and Meta Zimmeck (eds.), *Understanding the Roots of Voluntary Action: Historical Perspectives on Current Social Policy* (Brighton: Sussex Academic Press, 2011), pp. 82–94.

Thomson, Elaine, 'Between Separate Spheres: Medical Women, Moral Hygiene and the Edinburgh Hospital for Women and Children' in Steve Sturdy (ed.), *Medicine, Health and the Public Sphere in Britain 1600–2000* (London: Routledge, 2002), pp. 107–22.

Titmuss, Richard, *Problems of Social Policy* (London: HMSO, 1950).

Tout, Herbert, *The Standard of Living in Bristol* (Bristol: University of Bristol/ Arrowsmith, 1938).

Waddington, Keir, 'Unsuitable Cases: The Debate over Outpatient Admissions, the Medical Profession and Late-Victorian London Hospitals', *Medical History*, 42:1 (1998), 26–46.

Waddington, Keir, *Charity and the London Hospital, 1850–1898* (Woodbridge: Boydell Press, 2000).

Waddington, Keir, 'Paying for the Sick Poor: Financing Medicine under the Victorian Poor Law: The Case of the Whitechapel Union, 1850–1900' in Martin Gorsky and Sally Sheard (eds), *Financing Medicine: The British Experience since 1750* (London: Routledge, 2006), pp. 95–111.

Ward, Stephanie, 'The Means Test and the Unemployed in South Wales and the North-East of England, 1931–1939', *Labour History Review*, 74:1 (2008), 113–32.

Wardley, Peter (ed.), *Bristol Historical Resource*, CD-ROM (Bristol: University of the West of England, 2001).

Webster, Charles, *The Health Services since the War, Volume 1: Problems of Health Care, The National Health Service Before 1957* (London: HMSO, 1988).

Webster, Charles, 'Conflict and Consensus: Explaining the British Health Service', *Twentieth Century British History*, 1:2 (1990), 115–51.

Webster, Charles, *The National Health Service: A Political History*, 2nd revised edition (Oxford: Oxford University Press, 2002).

Weindling, Paul (ed.), *Healthcare in Private and Public from the Early Modern Period to 2000* (London: Routledge, 2015).

Willis, Tim, 'The Bradford Municipal Hospital Experiment of 1920: The Emergence of the Mixed Economy in Hospital Provision in Inter-War Britain' in Martin Gorsky and Sally Sheard (eds), *Financing Medicine: The British Experience since 1750* (London: Routledge, 2006), pp. 130–44.

Willmott, Phyllis, '1895–1945: The First 50 Years' in Joan Baraclough, Grace Dedman, Hazel Osborn and Phyllis Willmott (eds), *100 Years of Health Related Social Work 1895–1995: Then – Now – Onwards* (Birmingham: British Association of Social Workers, 1996), pp. 1–11.

Woodward, John, *To Do the Sick No Harm: A Study of the British Voluntary Hospital System to 1875* (London: Routledge and Kegan Paul, 1974).

Zelizer, Viviana A., *The Social Meaning of Money: Pin Money, Paychecks, Poor Relief, and Other Currencies* (New York: Princeton University Press, 1994).

Index